- JEAN-MICHEL BOUDARD -

STRETCH EXERCISES FOR HORSES

BUILD AND PRESERVE MOBILITY, STRENGTH, AND SUPPLENESS

Translated by Elizabeth Gray

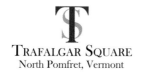

TRAFALGAR SQUARE
North Pomfret, Vermont

First published in the United States of America
in 2022 by Trafalgar Square Books
North Pomfret, Vermont 05053

Originally published in French as *Le stretching pour votre cheval.*

ISBN: 978-1-64601-093-6
Library of Congress Control Number: 2021949929

Photography: © Jean-Michel Boudard
Illustrations: © Marine Oussedik
Cover design: RM Didier
Translation into English: Elizabeth Gray
Index by Andrea M. Jones (www.jonesliteraryservices.com)

Printed in China

10 9 8 7 6 5 4 3 2 1

CONTENTS

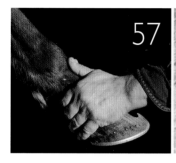 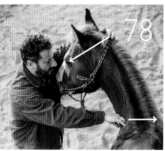 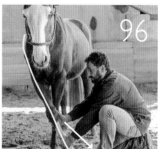

PREFACE

Jean-Michel Boudard's work in this book goes far beyond the framework of the usual advice to riders that reappears periodically in print, repeating the same evidence and presenting the same conclusions in various forms. Within it, I made genuine discoveries, with clear and precise concepts that have never, to my knowledge, been offered before to anyone who wants to give their horse an edge.

The many riders who wish to combine success in horse sport and the well-being of their mount are faced with a persistent dilemma: They can't help but feel that these two objectives are mutually exclusive....

Attempting to resolve this problem by facilitating work through the administration of analgesics is a double error—the products that can be used in this manner are prohibited in competition, and, more importantly, they do not prevent the horse's body from breaking down physically. Quite the contrary, in fact. The horse goes beyond his limits, unable to feel himself pass them, and wear-and-tear on the joints and internal organs is accelerated.

The only real solution is to reduce the discomfort of the animal legitimately, rather than attempt to hide it. Athletes are not able to work at their maximum potential every single day; efforts must be made to allow them to exercise their skill to a degree as close as possible to that ideal. There is no method of training or care that will allow a horse to perform at 110% of his capacity.

Here, you'll find a simple and effective way to minimize the biomechanical obstacles hampering a horse, while making his work both easier and more enjoyable.

Indeed, not only will his muscles and joints become less restricted, his natural movements will become more ample.

You won't exceed your horse's limits—you'll find you've expanded them. A pain-free horse who delights in his work performs better. You'll also delay the onset of age-related disorders.

This stretching procedure has been known and practiced by human athletes for a long time. Jean-Michel deserves every praise for adapting it to horses. The comparisons he uses to explain it, such as when he draws an analogy to a system of interconnected cogs, are easily understood by all, and require no background in biomechanics or physiology that would extend beyond the scope of this book.

Another appreciable advantage of the technique he offers us is that it will improve the relationship you have with your horse: You'll make him feel better with your own two hands. You'll establish a connection that goes beyond riding and, above all, you'll become aware, through this technique, of your horse's physical limits. This will help you learn to feel how far you can rightly ask him to push himself, without an injury during competition to make it clear to you.

Prevention is better than cure, as they say—but too few people give this saying the credence it deserves. To prevent problems before they can occur, that's the real goal, and this book is a major key to achieving it.

Dominique GINIAUX,
veterinary doctor and osteopath

INTRODUCTION

For more than thirty years, I have been interested in athletic pursuits and their impact on the body.

Sports are said to be good for our health, so why do they cause so many physical problems? This question has dogged me since I swam competitively at high intensity as a teenager, to the point where I was preparing for the French national student championships. Powerful spinal pain due to my physical growth at the time, an unbalanced diet that caused deficiencies, and an ill-suited training program forced me to end all participation in sports to avoid chronic joint degeneration. It brought my plans to become a physical education instructor to a premature end. From then on, I decided I wanted to address athletes' health instead!

After obtaining a diploma in massage therapy, I underwent additional studies at the French National Institute of Sport, Expertise, and Performance (INSEP) and very quickly became attached to a Parisian team that played American football, as well as to the French Swimming Federation, with which I worked for ten years. I was astounded to see firsthand the decrease in tendonitis, muscle sprains, and spinal blockages following the systematic application of stretching at each workout. During my first job as an assistant in the physiotherapy department for the French national judo team, I discovered an impressively effective technique: osteopathy. I immediately undertook a course of study that fascinated and even sometimes overwhelmed me. I am deeply grateful for the trust placed in me by the athletes, patients, and sports federations with whom I have worked. I was profoundly passionate about this new holistic way of approaching the care of the individual as a whole rather than any single pathology, of searching for and treating causes rather than symptoms, and of the excellent results it yielded.

On a personal level, following a regimen of osteopathy sessions and postural stretching, it was possible for me to resume normal activity without back pain; I even resumed playing sports. This experience was almost magical; I went from being unable to even swim to pursuing tennis, horseback riding, and the practice of equine osteopathy, a physical activity that I would argue demands effort comparable to a sport.

In this book, it is with the strongest conviction that I would like to share with you my method of equine stretching, so that it can become yours.

The most important advantage of this technique can be summed up in a few words: it is without risk for either the horse or rider, it can be practiced by anyone, and it is often complementary to osteopathic techniques and veterinary treatments. Learning to practice stretching with and for your horse will give you an independent and discerning understanding of biomechanical and behavioral problems.

Since 1996, I have been teaching my technique in France, across Europe, and in the United States, both to equine health professionals (including osteopaths, chiropractors, veterinarians, and acupuncturists) and to professional and amateur riders.

This third edition of the book captures my methodology as it has been improved by years of teaching, and the thousands of questions asked that have helped me refine the content and practice of my methods. The feedback has been unanimous: everyone discovers a complementary place for stretching in their daily routine.

What is stretching? Stretching is a form of physical exercise in which a specific muscle or muscle chain is deliberately flexed or extended in order to improve muscular elasticity and tone. Taking into account discoveries in neuromuscular physiology, stretching is a valuable therapeutic technique in its own right, approved in training centers for high-level athletes. Today, stretching is essential in all types of sports and athletic rehabilitation, allowing athletes to consistently improve their performance. It is a simple and effective technique, when applied in keeping with its fundamental principles.

When in competition, a horse's training places high demands on his body's systems (cardiovascular, muscular, articular, and nervous, to name a few) and requires deft technical ability on his part. Consequences: pain, strain, sprains, osteoarthritis, inflammation, and psycho-emotional dysfunctions that can slow down his training program, or even bring it to a halt entirely. As part of the care provided by the team that tends to him (trainer, barn attendant, farrier, veterinarian, osteopath, acupuncturist, and massage therapist), stretching can prevent many of these ailments. Daily stretching allows the athlete—including the equine athlete—to undertake a full work schedule while maintaining neuro-musculo-skeletal equilibrium, which is essential to fluidity of movement.

We know that any sports season is dependent on consistent performance: the more continuously an athlete is healthy and performing at their best, the more achievable their competitive objectives will be. This is what makes it essential to preserve the physical parameters of athletic performance, all of them closely linked: strength, flexibility, speed, coordination, and resilience. The practice of stretching makes it possible to maintain all these elements in harmony, in combination with a training program that includes phases of work and phases of rest and integration on physiological, energetic, and psycho-emotional levels.

An observation: a good number of horses spend twenty hours a day in their stalls and eat two or three meals. This schedule, imposed on them by humans, does not actually suit their physiology. This is why developing a means to compensate for that kind of inconsistency between physiology and treatment seems to me to be the least we can do for our equine friends. A rider asks his horse, after spending hours in his stall, to be ready to run and jump as soon as the rider arrives, when the rider herself wouldn't even think of running half a mile, over hurdles, the instant she got out of bed! The enforced immobility and the tendency to try to roll around in a cramped stall increase the risk of joints stiffening or locking; the horse will naturally attempt to deal with this by stretching on his own as best he can.

There is an important point that has been demonstrated to me on a daily basis by my osteopathic practice. Vital internal energies are much stronger in animals that live in a natural environment than in those that live in stalls and then go out for a short time to a closed arena or training course. In addition to the lack of space, and thereby of free movement so essential to the optimal functioning of physiological and mental bodily systems, many competition horses lack social time spent with other horses. Even the lack of a seasonally diverse diet for horses with no access to pasture can affect their internal energy. If we offer our horses the means to self-regulate in a natural setting, they will return the favor a hundred times over.

When I first approached applying osteopathy to horses on the competitive circuit, I was very surprised that the practice of stretching was not widespread, with the exception of a few stables that practiced muscle extension in an experimental way. I then recommended that trainers stretch all horses at least once a day, focusing on specific muscle chains, and especially those related to the issues which had brought me there. Following my recommendations quickly resulted in remarkable success.

Stretching must become an essential healing and preparation technique for the horse, in addition to warming up before work, active recovery after work, massage, and all other care given to the horse (food supplements, vitamins, trace elements ...) outside of actual training. Stretching will allow the animal to re-harmonize, to work through and eliminate the various joint and muscle compensations he uses to deal with life in his stall.

Stretching is a complementary technique that cannot be used in place of a veterinary checkup. It will not allow you to make medical diagnoses; that is reserved for your horse's veterinary team, with all their scientific knowledge and means of examination. As a preventative and curative technique, however, it does have the advantage of working effectively without chemical intervention. It is a valuable link between veterinary care and the act of riding.

The first section of this book is devoted to a simplified explanation of the anatomical and physiological basis for understanding the principles of stretching. It will then be easier to grasp the effects of muscle tension on gait and behavior. You will also find a description of my "neuro-muscular stretching" method—it is different in its physiological underpinnings from the stretching methods of other practitioners you may have encountered. I provide the details necessary to put it into practice immediately (simple, quick-to-perform evaluations, how to apply stretching to specific muscle chains, relaxation, preparation for work, recovery, and training of the young horse). I will then share the indications and contraindications.

The second section is oriented toward the visual. Photographs of each of the joint evaluation sequences capture each step, described in detail in the accompanying text (axes of movement, amplitude of movement, how to carry out evaluations on the fore-legs versus the hind legs versus the spine), with explanations of evaluations for entire muscle chains to allow you to decide which stretch and which orientation will serve your horse the most effectively.

Do not forget that stretching is also a privileged moment of connection between horse and rider; the rider must listen to her horse's body, without the constraints of obedience or force.

This creates a relationship of trust. It's an excellent way for trainers to help their students access certain analytical skills and learn how to work with their horses. And any rider's equitation will only improve as a result.

May this book make you want to put your hands on your horse: to feel him, to listen to him, and to understand him, in ways only the body comprehends.

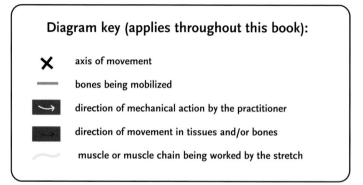

Diagram key (applies throughout this book):

✗   axis of movement

—   bones being mobilized

↪   direction of mechanical action by the practitioner

↪   direction of movement in tissues and/or bones

～   muscle or muscle chain being worked by the stretch

CHAPTER 1

FUNCTIONAL ANATOMY AND PHYSIOLOGY

A holistic view of health and disease

Here is a holistic look at the way the horse is put together. We begin with the physical body, which is animated by energy. This living body feels desires and emotions on one level, and it thinks, reflects, and remembers on another (the mind). These are interdependent: a physical problem can create an energetic, emotional, or mental imbalance in the horse. A change on any level requires an adjustment on each of the others. All of this must be considered without losing sight of the fact that these four components—physical, energetic, emotional, and mental—form a whole. Like many animals, horses have a higher level of awareness than humans. The horse interprets environmental data around him (the ground beneath his hooves, other creatures who are sharing his space, whether he has entered a space that will have a "positive" or possibly "negative" effect on him), as well as human intentions, by "decoding" the surrounding information and energy. He will then naturally put himself in a position where he is able to recharge his own internal energy.

✦ The physical body

The physical body is the tangible structure of the horse's form, including all biological systems: musculoskeletal, digestive, nervous, endocrine, immune, respiratory, circulatory, lymphatic, excretory, and reproductive—and also the organization of the fascia surrounding and protecting each of these configurations.

✦ Energy

Energy animates matter by giving it life, stimulating each cell to function in its specific role. It manifests via the rhythms and frequencies specific to each biological system (circulatory, lymphatic, respiratory, etc). These rhythms adapt based on other rhythms:

- exterior (rhythm of life, cycle of the seasons, etc.)

- interior (the body is regulated by various "biological clocks," and research regularly discovers new kinds of biological cycles. All bodily systems are animated by their own rhythms, which can change depending on many parameters such as emotional state, time of day, degree of physical activity, etc.)

All these rhythms of life are governed by the principle of homeostasis (from the Greek *homeo:* "alike; the same," and *stasis:* "standing still; unchanging"), which applies to all the regulatory processes maintaining biological balance in any living being. This self-regulating capacity for internal maintenance presupposes sufficient vitality. That vitality comes from different sources of energy: the vital energy possessed at birth; the energy supplied by food, respiration, psycho-emotional and social balance; the energy exchanged by animals with each other, or with places, plants, or humans; and the energy of physical exercise.

Osteopathic theory suggests that maintaining good health requires the proper management of all these types and sources of energy.

It follows that a horse with low energy or insufficient vitality cannot be cared for in the same way as a horse with full vitality. Any stimulating technique that requires a response from the body's own energy cannot be used in the former case. An osteopathic therapist should therefore be trained to check a horse's energy state before attempting any treatment.

✦ Emotions

The horse feels emotions (fear, joy, desire, anger), which have an influence on the function of his body's systems. Consider, for example, a frightened horse: his muscles tense up, his focus narrows to whatever is frightening him. Another example: a horse in training loses morale; his ears are held low, and he loses his appetite and fails to finish his meals.

The emotional plane is effectively linked to the history of the horse, to all the emotionally impactful moments he has experienced: birth, early training, any painful injuries or fights. The search for emotional balance is also connected to the horse's social environment. The emotional balance of a horse turned out to pasture with a bunch of his friends and the emotional balance of a horse shut up in his stall, except when he goes out once or twice a day to work, are not comparable.

There are two types of social environment:

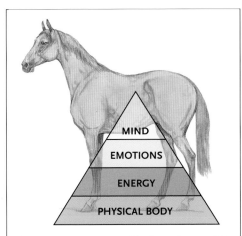

This holistic assessment of the horse is essential to understanding him. Indeed, it is only beginning with a big-picture view that will allow us to pinpoint the specific level on which the horse needs to be helped.

- human—with the groom, the rider, the trainer, the owner, the veterinary team.

- animal—with the horse's training partners, his family line, familiar horses of the opposite sex, members of his group or herd at the stable and the dominance dynamics that entails, even attachment to a barn animal of another species, etc.

The horse is very emotional. Any change in the behavior of his social companions will upset his balance, one way or another.

However, this also means that changing any one parameter of his social environment may potentially be the gateway to solving a problem.

✦ The mind and thoughts

A level with much weaker influence in the horse than in humans. The horse is a much more instinctive animal, but his conditioning at the hands of humans sometimes leads him to think a little too much. It's not uncommon for horses to be depressed—to do their jobs solely to please, out of duty rather than because they want to. When you look at these horses, there's a spark missing from their eyes. The causes are multiple, and can come from any or all of the levels mentioned. It's common to see a horse undergo a kind of metamorphosis when he's restored to a social environment with good friends. This reconnects him with his natural, unconditioned "core program." "He's got his head in the game again," say the trainers. Diversification of exercises and activities can also contribute to mental renewal.

The musculoskeletal system

✦ Bones

The skeleton is a support structure formed by the bones. Bone, a very dense and strong tissue, plays the role of stable understructure for the rest of the body. The bones are the fixed points to which tendons, muscles, ligaments, and other tissues attach themselves. Despite its great rigidity, bone tissue does have a capacity for intra-osseous movement, which, during intense effort, can help prevent the bone from fracturing. It's also a considerable reserve of minerals for the body (especially calcium, regulated by the secretions of the thyroid and parathyroids). Bone tissue is involved in the production of blood cells, via bone marrow. Cellular acidosis causes a drop in bone calcium concentration.

✦ Joints

The joints allow individual bones or groups of bones to move. The surfaces of joints are covered with cartilage and surrounded by a fibrous sleeve: the joint capsule. The joint capsule's fibrous structure, reinforced by ligaments, protects the joint by limiting its movement mechanically. It is lined with tissue that produces synovial fluid and contains a high concentration of nerves, receptors that give the nervous system a lot of information.

During movement, the joint surfaces slide over each other. The cartilage, which promotes this sliding, is nourished by synovial fluid (viscous, lubricating fluid inside the joint) and contains neither blood vessels nor nerves. Joint cartilage is able to absorb shocks well, thanks to the proteoglycan molecules it contains. It has the ability to hydrate itself when at rest, and to dehydrate under force or weight.

JOINT (CROSS-SECTION)

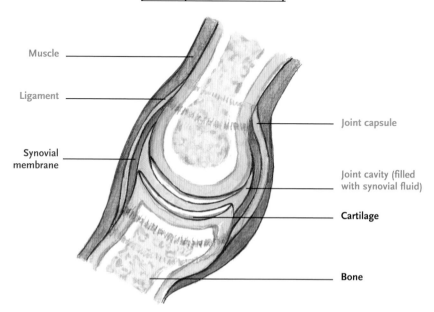

Muscle

Ligament

Synovial membrane

Joint capsule

Joint cavity (filled with synovial fluid)

Cartilage

Bone

A joint may swell as a result of:

- training or performance requests the horse cannot fulfill, bad balance, hard work on delicate hooves, hyperpressure on the joint due to muscular contraction or joint retraction (if older lesions or injuries to the joint are involved) following a stress on the joint, a fall, or a locking of the joint. An ensuing overproduction of synovial fluid will make the joint swell, and potentially become painful;

- a direct blow or wound;

- an excess of acidic or lipidic metabolic waste.

Each bone is connected to another by ligaments, which protect joints and hold them together.

These ligaments are the tissues damaged by a sprain or dislocation, when joint movement has not been properly controlled. The joints, when not in use (in cases of immobilization following trauma, or in old age), tend toward stiffness and fibrosis. They gradually lose their mobility, and end up locking up.

An increase in tone in the muscles surrounding a bone or joint increases the mechanical resistance of the bone or strengthens the joint. If the muscle is flexible, it also absorbs the vibratory forces of impacts against the ground.

The joints are mobilized by the muscles.

✦ Muscles

The muscles are attached to the bones by tendons, and wrap around the joints. They represent 60% of the total body weight. They move the articulated structure of the skeleton and ensure its stability, like rigging joining the masts and spars of a ship. The properties of muscle tissue are:

- elasticity (it returns to its initial shape after stretching);

- contractility (it shortens its fibers after a stimulus);

- excitability (it reacts to stimuli);

- extensibility (it can elongate as well as contract).

A muscle is made up of many fibers arranged in bundles, which are themselves grouped into larger bundles. Each of these bundles is surrounded by an envelope of connective tissue (fascia), partitioning the fibers of the same muscle, where the blood vessels and the network of nerves necessary for the muscles' proper function travel.

Looking at a muscle under a microscope would show us an entanglement of muscle fibers (myofilaments) arranged side by side. These can slide over each other. As shown in the diagram below, muscle fibers adapt to various stresses by sliding

MYOFILAMENT DIAGRAM

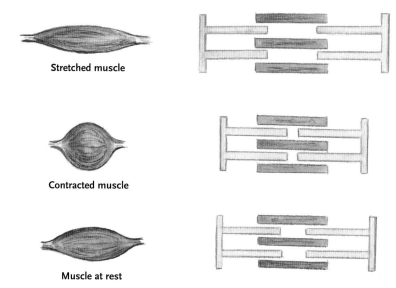

Stretched muscle

Contracted muscle

Muscle at rest

Muscle fibers slide over each other to greater or lesser degrees, depending on the muscle's state of tension.

in an interlacing fashion. If we start from a position of equilibrium with the muscle at rest:

- during a muscle contraction, muscle fibers tighten by sliding between each other, shortening and thickening the muscular body;

- when stretching, the myofilaments move apart—the muscle lengthens and decreases in diameter.

Stretching facilitates the sliding of muscle fibers and improves the elasticity of musculotendinous tissue. When you stimulate a contraction in a stretched muscle chain, you strengthen its ability to protect underlying joints in extreme postures. The brain gradually integrates information from these experiences by associating them with well-being, and the horse will thus be able to increase his mobility and awareness, thanks to an improved physical understanding of his own body.

Contraction of a muscle, the movement of sliding myofilaments, requires energy. Depending on the type of muscle, the work, and the level of training, the muscle may instead use oxygen, or the energy reserves provided by the breakdown of glycogen (sugar). When all these reserves have been used up, muscle tissue can also break down fat to synthesize energy.

There are two types of muscle function, corresponding to different anatomical groups:

* tonic—these are short muscles close to the joints, which maintain postural tone. They support joint structure in a favorable position for joint integrity, in order to protect the joints during powerful contractions of dynamic muscles. Tonic muscles are positioned deep down and close to joints, are very powerful since they work continuously, and are richly supplied with nerves and blood vessels. They're slow to contract, and mainly run on oxygen.

* dynamic—these are larger, more superficial muscles, which are used for dynamic movement of the body. They can provide strong, explosive contractions and are necessary for sport. They are fast but less powerful, and use oxygen and stored energy reserves during resting phases. These muscles gain volume and increase their energy capacity through training.

Balance is a continuous, reflexive adjustment in muscle tone.

Muscle has two types of sensory receptors designed to inform the brain of the position and stretch rate of muscle fibers. These receptors thus warn the control system of potential stretching or tearing.

There are two types of receptors:

* Golgi receptors, located at the myotendon junction; these receptors are stimulated by either stretching or contraction of the muscle.

* the neuromuscular spindle, located between the muscle fibers; these receptors are stimulated only by stretching of the muscle.

When a muscle is stretched, both types of receptors send a stimulus that will trigger a reflex arc through the spinal cord, creating a reflex contraction of that muscle (myotatic reflex). These receptors may be more or less sensitive depending on the temperature, the degree of physical and mental tension in the horse, and the rate of stretching.

Skin receptors and environmental and emotional context also play a role in adjusting the postural tone of the horse.

The principles of stretching derive from this neurophysiological data:

* warm up the muscle before stretching it;

* proceed gradually so as not to trigger muscle defense;

* hold for more than 6 to 8 seconds to decrease the triggering threshold of the muscle's defensive reflexes;

* work in a place that is calm and reassuring for the horse.

MUSCLE TONE REGULATION

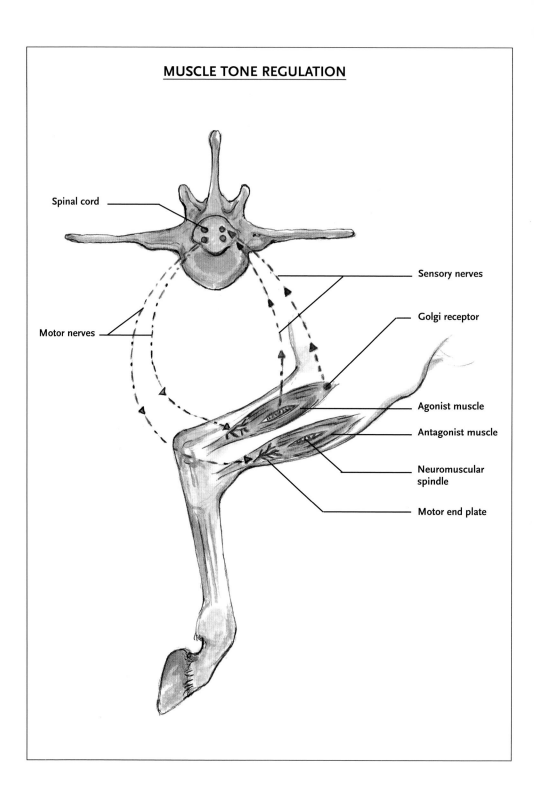

Spinal cord

Motor nerves

Sensory nerves

Golgi receptor

Agonist muscle

Antagonist muscle

Neuromuscular
spindle

Motor end plate

✦ The nervous system

The nervous system controls the skeletal muscles in two ways: the first way is voluntary, which is to say the horse decides to produce a movement. The second is the control of postural tone—an involuntary series of adjustments in the tone of supporting muscles, depending on the information that different receptors send to the brain. Receptors are found in the muscles, in the tendons of the muscles, in the ligaments, and on the skin.

They inform the central nervous system of the positions of the joints, the speed of joint movements, their amplitudes, and the degree of stretching in the muscle fibers.

Stretching, by stimulating muscle, joint, and skin receptors, sends information to the cortex and gradually reprograms the release of defensive muscle tension. It stimulates better concentration in the horse and an expansion in the scope of motor and body patterns, by asking for unusual movements.

THE PATH OF INFORMATION THROUGH THE NERVOUS SYSTEM

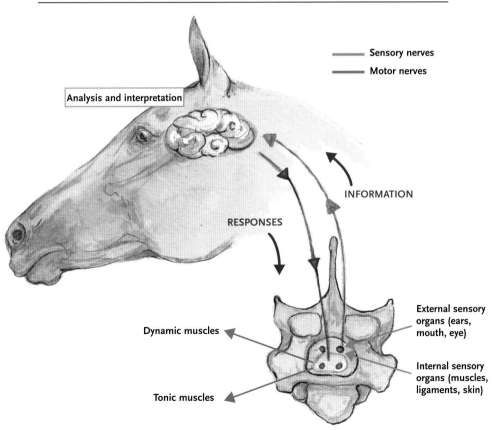

Sensory nerves

Motor nerves

Analysis and interpretation

INFORMATION

RESPONSES

Dynamic muscles

Tonic muscles

External sensory organs (ears, mouth, eye)

Internal sensory organs (muscles, ligaments, skin)

Postural tone, according to pioneering kinesiotherapist Boris Dolto, is "the slight contractile tension in which all normal skeletal muscle not directly engaged in a specific activity is found at all times, when it is at rest." Postural tone is regulated by the information given by the neuromuscular spindle, readjusted by the motor cell of the spinal cord, which is itself controlled by the medulla oblongata. (The medulla oblongata is the lowest part of the brain. It plays a critical role in transmitting signals between the spinal cord and the higher parts of the brain.) Postural tone also reflects the mental and emotional state of the horse in relation to his immediate environment. So when he is anxious, his degree of tone and overall tension increases.

Experience shows that the practice of stretching, by regularly shifting the horse's tissues into a state of relaxation, makes the horse less anxious. This demonstrates that physical techniques can act upon and change the behavior of a horse.

The autonomic system

The autonomic nervous system operates in parallel with the somatic or voluntary nervous system; as the name suggests, it functions autonomously. Not governed by individual, conscious decision-making, it controls visceral and glandular functions and can affect the mental and emotional state through the release of hormones.

It is made up of two complementary systems:

• the sympathetic system, which manages active reflexes such as "fight or flight"

• the parasympathetic system, which manages repair, regeneration of tissues, and procreative functions

Stress is a frequent source of disjunction between these systems, and causes symptoms such as aggressiveness, sadness, stomach pain, and disturbed heart rhythms. There is an interaction between the dysfunctions of structures innervated by the central nervous system and certain structures (viscera, vessels and skin) innervated by the autonomic nervous system. This can create a hyperexcitability that causes contraction of the muscles, with an accompanying decrease in joint mobility that osteopaths recognize as an "osteopathic lesion," often associated with visceral, vascular, and skin dysfunctions. This connection, and the potential for dysfunction, goes both ways.

Stretching re-harmonizes these two systems by mobilizing and releasing tension from the paravertebral and vertebral tissues where nerves pass.

✦ Fascia

New findings on fascia show that it is made of microfibrils rich in sensory receptors that connect the surface of the skin to the deepest areas of the body. They form contractile fibrous tissues surrounded by extra-cellular fluid, which themselves surround and internally penetrate all structures, and are also able to slide along those

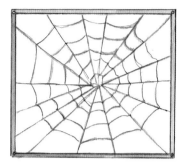
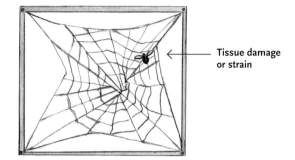

Tissue damage or strain

structures (including joint capsules, ligaments around the joints, periosteum around the bone, peritoneum around the viscera, aponeurosis around the muscles, connective tissue around the blood and lymphatic vessels, meninges around the nervous system, between the skin and the subcutaneous structures).

According to J.-C. Guimberteau, surgeon and researcher studying fascia, "tissue continuity guarantees functional unity thanks to the maintenance of body shape and its integrity." The fasciae are connected to each other, their fibrillar architecture allows maximum internal mobility of each organ in all directions, and they can adapt by reshaping themselves to deal with any constraints imposed by the body. They constitute a link that's mechanical, informational, and reflexive between all parts of the body, and can transmit pain and react to emotional states through piezoelectric stases or fixations.

Any problem related to any part of the body can generate, through these links of fascia, a repercussion of compensatory action throughout the whole body.

To understand the effect of tensions of the fascia on the horse's body, imagine a spider's web with homogenous, balanced thread tension. If you touch or hang a weight on a part of the web, however, a deformation of its shape and interior structure will occur, due to the sudden increase in tension on some of the threads. A system of adaptive, compensatory tension will then spread through all the threads of this spider's web, simply because they are connected to each other.

This notion of tissue organization is essential in the practice and understanding of stretching. It is in fact a sensitive reading of the tissues that must guide us in a particular direction with stretching. Until a knot or other strain in a muscle is resolved, the tissues affected by it will point us in its direction with their compensatory tension.

This posture corresponds to the posture of the horse during the trauma that caused the original problem. This is where the importance of properly caring for scars and, above all, their adhesions, no matter how small, becomes clear. Stretching facilitates sliding between the different layers of connective tissue by limiting friction. Resistance is thus reduced, and the gait of the horse is fuller and more relaxed.

A release of tension from fascia will often be associated with the disappearance of pain, and can also be the source of an emotional release that I encounter very frequently when treating horses.

The technique required to free the fascia consists of making contact with the tissues, and moving with them in the direction of ease of movement. The tissues use this contact and support to free themselves. During treatment with my neuromuscular stretching technique, we use the same principle of regulation.

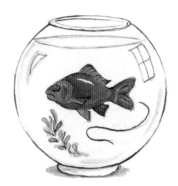 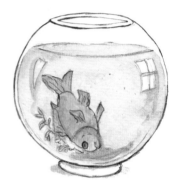

The cell as a functional unit of the horse's body

Every individual cell in a horse's body bathes in interstitial (or extra-cellular) nutrient fluid, and nourishes itself there by exchange through its membrane.

The heartbeat pushes arterial blood through blood vessels, delivering oxygen and nutrients to each cell in the body. The oxygenation of the blood takes place in the lungs, and the richness of blood nutrients depends on a good diet and good digestion.

Whatever their specific location and function (muscle, liver, skin, etc.), cells produce waste. This waste will be drained by the venous system and the lymphatic system, then filtered during passage through the liver, kidneys, lungs, or skin, and then finally evacuated by the large intestine or bladder, with the waste-free blood returned to the heart to start a new circulatory cycle.

✦ Comparison with a fish in a bowl

Picture it: the fish is a cell, and the water in its bowl is the extra-cellular fluid.

If I ask you what it takes to keep the fish healthy, you will say to me, "An air pump to oxygenate the water, a filter to drain and remove its waste, food to keep it fed, and don't forget to change the water every now and then."

If one day you find that your fish is behaving strangely, or is not moving around in its bowl as usual, then the first thing you will do is verify that all the pumps and filters are working well and that nothing is missing.

It sounds obvious, but sometimes we tend to forget about all those simple things that sustain life. The body is like a fishbowl in which hundreds of millions of fish—cells—are swimming. Overall health depends on the proper function of every one of them, and that proper function in turn depends on a suitable balance of extracellular fluid.

Significant functional problems can be caused by small capillaries (arterioles and venules) being compressed or dysfunctional, and therefore no longer able to supply extracellular fluid, meaning the process of cell perfusion becomes derailed. Arterioles have a smooth muscular wall, the diameter of which is regulated by the autonomic nervous system. This is why it is so important to observe and touch tissues in order to detect poorly vascularized regions that are no longer permitting optimal function.

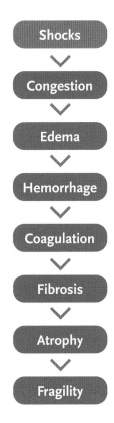

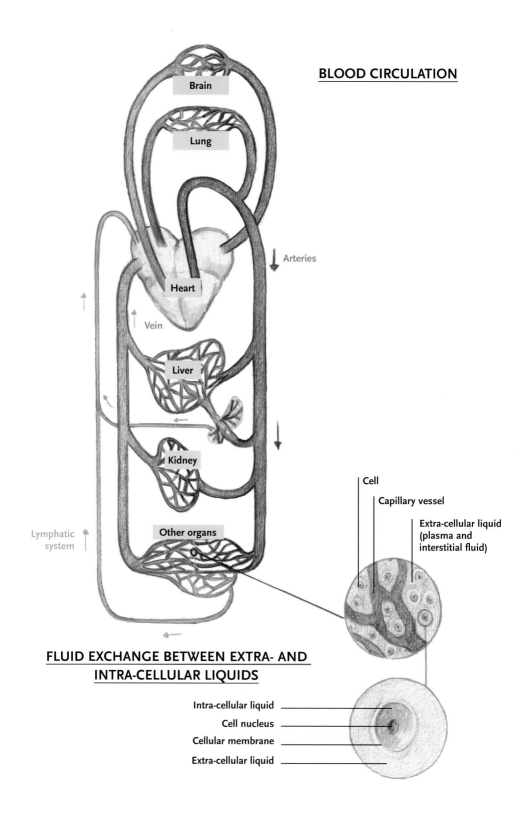

BLOOD CIRCULATION

Brain

Lung

Arteries

Heart

Vein

Liver

Kidney

Cell

Capillary vessel

Extra-cellular liquid
(plasma and
interstitial fluid)

Lymphatic
system

Other organs

**FLUID EXCHANGE BETWEEN EXTRA- AND
INTRA-CELLULAR LIQUIDS**

Intra-cellular liquid

Cell nucleus

Cellular membrane

Extra-cellular liquid

We find two types of problems at the cellular level:

- the cell is not receiving enough nutrients, which is referred to as a deficiency.

- the venous and lymphatic drainage system is not efficient and the cell is remaining loaded with waste, which results in toxicity at the level of the cell.

✦ Fragility of muscles or tendons

Thus, we can understand the progression of damage over time in the cells of a muscle or tendon undergoing trauma. This can be due to direct or indirect shocks, such as the vibratory resonance of the hooves impacting the ground. Whether the shocks are light and repeated, or singular but powerful, they cause congestion, then edema, between the cells. Blood may pass into the extra-cellular fluid (hemorrhage), which then will coagulate and cause the formation of fibrous tissue, reducing the elasticity of the muscle or tendon and promoting a lack of blood flow (ischemia). Oxygen deficiency and energy deficiency follow.

There is then degeneration of tissues, due to cell atrophy, and the development of muscle or tendon fragility. Areas experiencing hyperactivity are much hotter than areas experiencing hypoactivity, which can become completely cold; both have a consequence on our metaphorical balance sheet. Thermal testing is a reliable, fast, and inexpensive way to palpate and assess activity within an area of the body.

Stretching makes it possible to tackle the problem at its root by promoting movement, and the sliding of various tissues against each other. Tissue decongestion then occurs, and edema does not have time to set in. Along with massages and cold showers, stretching promotes the release of vasomotor constriction, and allows exchange at the cellular level to begin anew. Muscle tension is broken down, and the muscles regain their qualities of elasticity, contractility, and extensibility. The joints protected by these muscles become freer to move, too. Thus, the vicious cycle (pain > spasm > ischemia > retraction > pain) will be broken.

> *"Life is underpinned by the continual movement of liquids in cells and between cells. The slowing of these currents and exchanges is fatigue and illness, and their end is death."*
>
> (Dr Salmanoff, *Secrets et sagesse du corps*
> *[Secrets and wisdom of the body]*, Ed. La Table Ronde)

CHAPTER 2

POSTURE AND COMPENSATORY TENSION

Postural analysis

Analysis of the static posture of the horse when he's standing at rest on all four hooves shows us that he is more stable than a person is on two feet. Indeed, the horse's center of gravity is positioned between these four supports. Thanks to an anatomical peculiarity, the horse can sleep upright without muscular work by locking his kneecaps. He thus keeps his hind legs straight and positions himself in such a way as to find his balance.

Here is a little reminder from the physical sciences:

Balance is possible when the center of gravity is positioned between the points of support. If the horse projects his center of gravity backwards, that increases strain on the hindquarters. If the center of gravity ends up positioned more to one side than the other, the joints will be loaded asymmetrically.

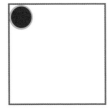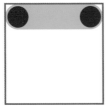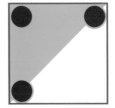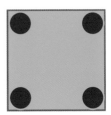

Center of gravity protection zones to maintain balance

During stretching, by accompanying the release of a muscle chain with the mobilization of a limb, for example, the practitioner can adjust the position of the horse's center of gravity along either axis (front-back and left-right). To ensure comfort in a balanced position, the horse modifies his postural tone in response to the information he receives. This means you can have a very precise and profound effect on the entire muscular support system, and on the entire spinal column, by working with the limbs (see tonic muscles).

Dynamic posture maintained at any gait or pace is the result of a succession of moments of unstable balance giving an appearance of fluidity. The posture changes to follow the gait of the horse. Riders sometimes talk about the "set" of the horse, as if we were programming his posture as we go. Thus, alternating between different gaits, especially for some very specialized horses such as trotters, would certainly be beneficial. Why not include sessions of galloping in a merry-go-round or jumping over small obstacles at liberty, which would maintain the horse's cardiovascular system, change the dynamic postural program, and break the vicious circle of very specific work-related muscle contractions repeating again and again? It would also be beneficial for the morale of the horse, who would take these sessions as a game.

Sensitive joint and muscle receptors provide information and allow adjustment and maintenance of balance both at rest and in motion.

The fluidity of a horse's gait depends on his physical structure, his level of energy, and the quality of his muscle condition.

Compensatory tension

The horse has an automatic physical organization system to adapt to movement while maintaining balance.

The body reacts in its entirety to any motion that risks disrupting its harmony. Any restriction in the mobility of a joint or the ability to stretch a muscle will be compensated for by other areas to allow function. This is the case with a horse observed to be more or less lame when cold, but whose symptoms of lameness fade as he is warmed up. This does not mean that the problem is solved, but rather that adaptation by the body made it possible to modify the angle or axis of one or more movements, in order to change the result and bypass any hindering forces.

To help you understand, imagine yourself walking or jogging with a little pebble in your shoe. You will feel discomfort with each step; the body will try to decrease the pain in your supporting limb by modifying your usual postural balance. This compensation will generate additional work for certain muscle chains. These muscle chains, not being used to doing their work in this way, will quickly tire and start to stiffen. That stiffness will spread to the pelvis, then along the spinal column to the cervical spine, thus "locking up" more and more areas, until the body can make no more compensatory adjustments.

The only solution the body can find to get out of this mess is an acute attack. It is not uncommon in such cases to have a stiff neck or experience back pain a few days later, from a small, harmless movement such as picking up a leaf from the floor or getting out of your bathtub.

If we observe a healthy horse that is well balanced in his locomotion, we will see that his movements are fluid and efficient. (Note in passing that even in these optimal conditions, some horses will not run as fast or jump as high as others.) We can say that he is performing to the best of his ability.

Let's imagine that this well-balanced horse has a joint problem, a muscle problem, or even a flesh wound. In order to avoid pain, a whole series of compensations will be put in place. Initially, the compensation will be local, confined to the area around the point that hurts. But very soon those initial compensations will become painful in their turn, and the whole body will look for a better "solution." At this initial stage, the problem and accompanying compensation sometimes go unnoticed in the horse's movement, as if the degree of difficulty due to the underlying problem has been diluted, dispersed throughout the body. Not all horses are equal at this level of injury. In fact, horses with very flexible tissues ("eel" types) will not show any signs at all, whereas a horse with stiffer tissues will not be able to compensate, or will be able to compensate only a little, and will begin to suffer more obviously more quickly from relatively small osteopathic lesions.

Let's move forward in time ...

The horse is worked as if nothing had happened. Every possible avenue of compensation is sought desperately. The body requisitions the dynamic muscles, whose function is to contract for explosive movements, and uses them to maintain a defensive posture instead. As we saw in Chapter 1 (see p. 11), the physiology of those muscles is not suitable for this kind of work. Very quickly, they will become painful. This will lead to muscle strain and inflammation of the joints due to overexertion. The horse will start to limp, or he will change his behavior. There is no point in increasing constraints in an effort to prevent the horse from expressing his discomfort; this only displaces the problem and increases the risk of reluctance. Now is the right time for the rider or trainer to decide to treat the real issue and seek to understand the causes of this locomotive and behavioral change.

In my osteopathic practice, the true question is locating the cause of the cause of the problem. In a limping horse with many sore spots, where did the issues originally start? It's not easy to resolve problems when they stack up. Secondary osteopathic lesions become primary over time, especially if the same activity is repeated increasingly often.

One of the laws of osteopathy should never be forgotten: "Anything can affect everything." For many riders, the back seems to be essential to their reading of the horse. In fact, musculo-vertebral pain can be the body's expression of a dysfunction, like a light bulb that starts blinking to say something needs to change. Osteopathic reasoning aims to look for the seed cause of the problem.

The osteopath looks for areas and tissues that are restricted in movement and that may or may not be painful through a basic assessment. It's possible that most of the areas examined will be painful on palpation, and often hot from overexertion of the underlying muscle. It is possible to put an analgesic or an anti-inflammatory that will give the impression of having solved the problem. The real question is: why was this area working so hard that it became inflamed and painful? My daily practice shows that it suffices to revive rigid areas, which are often cold with disuse on palpation, to decrease the work of the rest and thereby reduce inflammation and pain. I am not saying that we shouldn't help the painful, inflamed areas, but that the results of treatment clearly last longer when the treatment is focused on reviving "locked-up" areas and resolving stiffness in tissue. A dysfunction somewhere in the limbs can, through compensatory tensions, lock up part of the back—and, in turn, the dysfunctions of the back can generate compensations that run down the limbs.

BALANCED TENSION

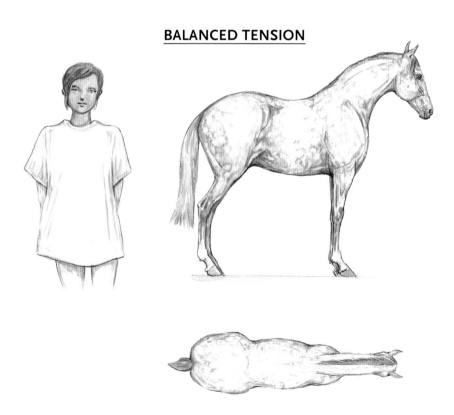

THE START OF A CHAIN OF COMPENSATIONS

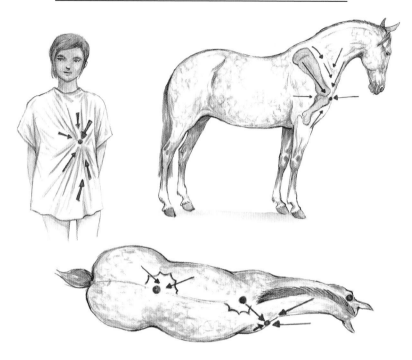

By practicing stretching, you can detect the problem in its earliest stages, without letting its momentum get away from you; it's the best solution for the horse, the rider, and your budget. Studies have shown that regular maintenance of sound horses reduces the cost of more intensive care such as systemic anti-inflammatories to extinguish a full-blown crisis in a limited time, or injections for anything that is painful (with resulting delays to allow the drugs to pass through the horse's system in time for competition), or to handle any area that seems blocked. Everything is possible; everything has its symptoms and its consequences.

A daily stretching session allows you to spot problems in their early stages. It is preventive. It is then up to you to make the choice of how to solve the problems once they've been detected.

In the diagram above, we took the example of a horse with a problem in the front of his right shoulder. Whatever the origin, this restriction of mobility will initially hamper the area near the shoulder. Then the whole body will seek to adapt its posture to maintain balance during the work required of the horse, in order to absorb the discomfort of this restriction of shoulder mobility.

In this case, the problem in the front of the shoulder will hamper the extension of the right foreleg—and yet, once the horse is warmed up, discomfort will no longer be visible. Very quickly, with work, the compensations will progress deeper. We can typically find painful tension in the lower right cervical muscles (right lateral tilt) and upper left cervical muscles (left lateral tilt, to keep the horse looking straight forward), along with tension in the left withers and lumbar spine.

Compensation could be compared to a rescue operation, useful in maintaining a minimum of function. Here we have a paradox: Mother Nature offers a rescue operation so as to ensure the minimum and prevent the body from running out of fuel while waiting for a solution to the initial problem. However, many riders struggle to deal with this minimum degree of function; they push, in the hope of achieving the previous non-minimum baseline of effective performance. This pressure overheats the system, so to speak.

The compensations become increasingly harmful through this over-straining, and the body is unable to reverse the process on its own.

Even the smallest area of knotted or strained tissue can disrupt the motor skills and body synchronization essential to a horse's performance.

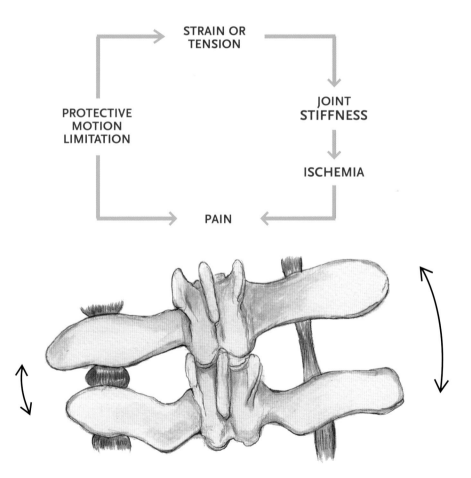

Joint contracture and stiffness, trigger point

In osteopathic practice, a "contracture" can be defined as a physiological response in a muscle to numerous stimuli in the course of various pathological processes: pain, inflammation, tissue degeneration, poor posture. Considered as a defensive reaction, sometimes it can, over time, exceed its goal and become more troublesome than the initial pathology—a vicious circle from which you must escape as quickly as possible.

A contracture in a muscle chain causes a reduction in range of motion (stiffness), which reduces the mobility of the tissues around a joint. There is then a decrease in cellular exchange due to lack of vascularization. The tissues become loaded with toxins, and become painful. This pain generates additional protective contractures, and the painful cycle continues.

In the diagram on the previous page, we can see, on the left, a contracture affecting the two vertebrae laterally and compressing the left hind joint. The muscle on the right side is then constantly stretched, along with the joint capsule on the same side. Any movement becomes difficult to achieve, and gradually the two vertebrae are "locked" by contractures.

While a contracture is, at the beginning, a useful reaction, once enough time has passed with the contracture in place, it becomes an obstacle to a good recovery for both joint and muscles. Its treatment is therefore imperative. When it has been present for a long time, in addition to treating the original cause of the contracture, it will be necessary to treat the consequence of the contracture: muscle fibrosis. The usual techniques are massage, joint manipulation, physiotherapy (heat or cold, shock waves, electrotherapy, magnotherapy), acupuncture, and mesotherapy.

In the long term, fibrous tissue can become necrotic. If regular work is continued in such a case, muscle fibrosis can progress to rupture of muscle fibers or a tendon, because the muscle tissue will have lost its elastic properties.

And if the contracture was helpful? Contractures are to be considered not problems to be eliminated, but red flags indicating there is another issue to watch out for. Indeed, once the originating problem or problems have been discovered and dealt with, the contracture will no longer be necessary to the body, and will release. If it persists, that means that a deeper problem than the one you've treated still exists (for example, a stress fracture or injury to a tendon at the point of insertion into the foot, both of which are potentially difficult to identify). Sometimes a contracture is the result of an emotional or behavioral problem. If the horse is generally hyper-tense, a contracture may be due to inflammatory dysfunction of the digestive system. A hormonal problem in a mare can cause tension and contractures all over the affected side, from the jaw to the shoulder, flank, and hindquarters, as well as under the belly and the sternum (this not an exhaustive list).

Trigger points or pressure points: this concept is described in humans as a point that projects pain, sometimes at a distance, when pressed. A precise mapping of these points and their associated pain has been established. Therapists using this method refer to a description of the location of the patient's pain, and then, based on this mapping, look for the associated point that's capable of triggering the described pain.

Once this verification is done, treatment is applied to the point through acupressure massage (pressing with the fingertip perpendicular to the surface of the skin, maintaining circular pressure for about one minute), with an acupuncture needle, or by injection, and the pain recedes. In the horse, no mapping has been done because the horse can't describe where else in the body he is feeling pain when we press on a point of tension.

Movement and resistance

To move, the horse mobilizes his joints with muscle contractions. The freer the range of motion in his joints, the easier all movements are to perform, and the less the muscles tire.

Moving a joint requires overcoming the weight of the bone or bones to be mobilized, through muscle contraction. Physiology dictates that during the contraction of

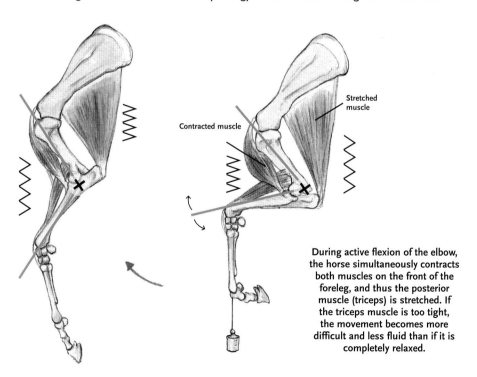

Stretched muscle

Contracted muscle

During active flexion of the elbow, the horse simultaneously contracts both muscles on the front of the foreleg, and thus the posterior muscle (triceps) is stretched. If the triceps muscle is too tight, the movement becomes more difficult and less fluid than if it is completely relaxed.

a muscle chain, there is an automatic relaxation of the opposing muscles which might otherwise slow or reverse the movement.

However, it can happen that the active muscle is forced to overcome both the weight of the bones and the resisting force of the opposing or antagonist muscles (which make the opposite movement when they contract).

Why are the antagonist muscles braking the movement?

Neurological problems aside, this unintended resistance can come from a contracture due to toxin overload, or stiffness caused by fibrosis of the antagonist muscle.

In equestrian disciplines, the search for performance often involves powerful take-offs. Muscle mass increases in volume from this kind of exercise, and often simultaneously loses flexibility. It then becomes a brake on any opposing muscles, increasing resistance to movement. It takes more muscle to gain the power to overcome that resistance, but more muscle would cause more resistance in its turn. Here we are again in another vicious circle.

The factors involved in performance on the locomotor level include, of course, muscle strength, but at the same time, there is a persistent need to lower the resistance of the muscles and improve the synchronization of movement. That way the horse will regain bounce and fluidity in his movements.

Stretching antagonist muscles lowers resistance to movement and relieves pressure on joints. With this technique, you can prevent premature wear and tear on the joints, decrease the onset of osteoarthritis, and fight inflammatory and degenerative effects on joint tissue.

✦ Stretch the limbs to free the back

During equine stretching training courses, I am always asked the same thing: "But the back, I want to learn techniques for the back..." (implied: "So when are we going to start working on the important things?"). As if all the problems come from the back.

When a light bulb won't turn on anymore in a room, the problem might, of course, be the bulb—but it might also be the switch, the wire carrying electricity to the bulb, or the fuse controlling the flow of electricity to the wire. The spine is even more complicated than a light bulb; it protects the entire nervous system. If there is dysfunction anywhere along the spine, it can cause peripheral pain, and the reverse is true: a tendon or joint in a dysfunctional limb can lock a spinal area, which in turn will become painful. This osteopathic lesion will be secondary to the limb problem; therefore, it is the limb that needs to be treated, and once that treatment is successful, spinal function will correct itself automatically.

We have learned in our overview of anatomy that the postural muscles allow the underlying architecture of the skeleton to be stable. The spine is in contact with the ground through the limbs, and the brain receives sensory information from receptors in the limbs. The brain analyzes and integrates the information it receives, and sends

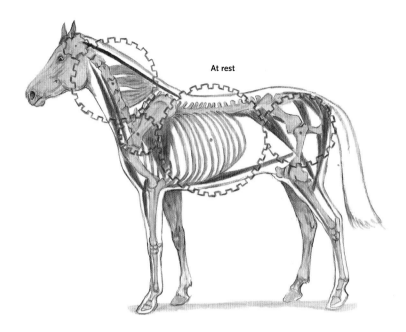

At rest

instructions for a postural adaptation to the back, according to the quality, amplitude, and speed of the body's movements. It is common for back pain occurring without a traumatic (fall, shock, blockage) or infectious cause to be due to hypercompensatory inflammation of another restricted area. That leaves one or more vertebrae crying out, "Help, I'm sick of doing all the work!" The solution is to give them a vacation, but also, and above all, to increase muscle length and range of motion in other areas, so that they no longer have to always compensate.

The same reasoning can apply to the forelimbs. The lengthening of the foreleg will promote a descent of the withers, and the reverse movement in the hind area will tend to lower the horse's head.

In the diagrams on the following page, we see the influence of a tension that ends up distributed across all the rest of the body. This prevents a lot of wear and even damage to certain structures of the musculoskeletal system. The explanation for many spinal pains can be given by these "cogs," and the way they distribute strain.

Take the example of a horse with retraction of the anterior muscles of the hind legs. These tensions prevent him from extending very far behind in his strides. To improve the range of motion for this extension, the lumbar vertebrae are forced to compensate with greater downward tilt mobility. Inflammation of the lower back is then inevitable, because the lumbar vertebrae are over-stressed. The muscles that surround this area are working at the limits of their physiology. They get tired, and very quickly the area becomes stiff and takes longer and longer to warm up. There is inflammation that will need to be treated in the spine—but until the flexor muscles gain length, that inflammation will never be gone for long.

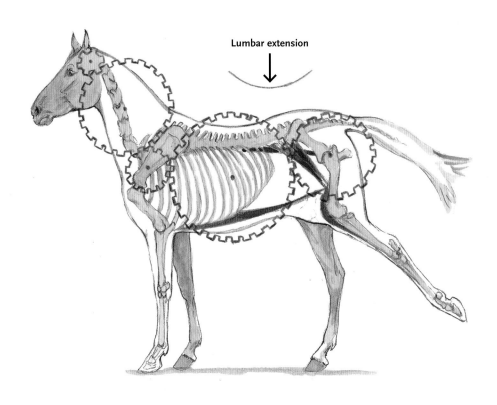

Lumbar extension

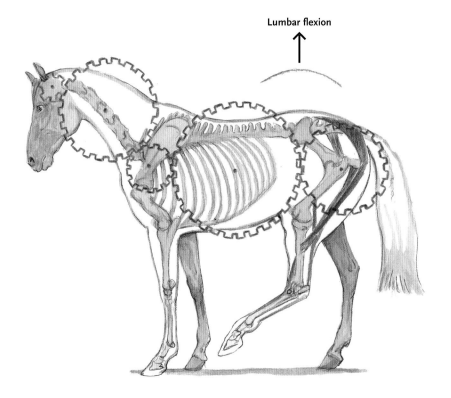

Lumbar flexion

Another frequently encountered example is pain in the withers with a sagging topline and sore paravertebral muscles. This horse will have a limitation in reach towards the front of the forelegs. When asked to lengthen his pace, the muscles of his forelegs tighten and pull on the withers, which try to compensate on the way down. The balance of tension is then upset, fatigue accumulates, and the vicious circle of contracture sets in.

In general, when tissue release is achieved correctly on a limb, that release extends through the entire spine. There will then be a change in postural tone throughout the body. Moreover, it is in keeping with osteopathic principle to exaggerate the adaptation pattern until a reaction of automatic self-correction is obtained. It's impressive to see the topline rebalance after ten minutes of stretching. This shows that we are changing the information reaching the postural system, which extends throughout the body without boundaries. All tissues are connected to each other, and any change in tension in one location causes change in all other tissues.

The balance of the back is a function of the tension ratio between the muscle tone of the superficial and deep abdominals (flexors) and that of the paravertebrals (extensors). A sagging back is held not by muscle tone, but by the osteoligamentary system. So when you ask for a longer gait, this movement pulls even more on the spine. When this request is painful, there is compensation, and when compensation is no longer possible, the horse rebels. This is his way of saying "Stop, I can't take it anymore!"

In this case, the role of stretching will be to release the tensions of the muscle chains connecting the limb to the spine. Particular care should be taken to obtain good length of the shoulder extensor muscles and hip flexor muscles.

It will remain for the rider to work at the same time on strengthening the abdominals during training in order to obtain commitment to the movement without causing pain to the horse.

The daily repetition of stretching sessions makes it possible to very quickly detect changes in the range of motion or reaction of the horse. When this is the case, we must immediately seek an explanation in order to intervene as quickly as possible. This allows for quick response, helping the horse's healthcare team diagnose and treat the issue before there is too much damage.

Advice

Always have a notebook for each horse. You can write down or draw the range of motion and degree of energy, any compensatory postural elements you notice, any defensive responses, locations of contractures, and locations of any wounds, with the date. This will allow you to follow the horse's progress over time.

Causes of pathology in the musculoskeletal system

✦ Biomechanical origins

- Static postural disorders such as bad balance, congenital deformities, or the after-effects of trauma. The farrier's role is especially important: with skilled trimming and suitable shoe fittings, these disorders can be compensated for.

- Muscle and tendon hypertension, permanent tightness that can hamper movement, premature wear and tear of the joints.

- Compensation for an untreated or poorly treated osteopathic lesion will generate secondary lesions, in a chain of interlinked compensations, until the horse is functionally immobilized because his body can no longer compensate at any level.

- Certain anti-symptomatic treatments which prevent compensation and do not treat the basic problem; the horse then works because he no longer feels any pain, but the problem remains.

- Changes of season and climate (dry cold vs wet cold, thunderstorms or windstorms, heat) have an influence on muscle tension.

- Poor agonist/antagonist ratios, which we know to increase the risk of breakdown (and which points to diversifying the horse's work and performing recommended stretches following exercise).

- Overwork and stress cause tissue acidity, which can lead to many symptoms.

✦ Biological origins

- A diet not suitable for the type or degree of work. This can clog tissues with toxins and cause acidosis from overeating or nutritional miscalculations.

- Toxic cellular overloads: the body must eliminate daily waste and toxins, either brought into the system from outside (additives and synthetic drugs, pollution), or originating within and produced by the body itself (waste from daily functioning). Elimination is provided by the excretory organs, including the kidneys, intestines, lungs, and skin. Intestines that are irritated (by bad daily habits, and causing bad digestion) for example, can produce an excess of toxic elements such as oxalic acid, which will, if it is not quickly eliminated, diffuse through the body, causing disease-like symptoms (arthritis attacks, outbreaks of skin irritation, nasopharyngeal inflammation attacks, etc).

- Deficiencies depriving the body of certain essential nutrients (trace elements, vitamins).

- Poor hydration. You should know that water is a major element in the constitution of the horse's body; it makes up 75% to 80% of his weight. It is therefore essential to ensure a good supply in terms of both quality and quantity.

- Infections and inflammations (ears-nose-throat, pulmonary, urinary infection; chronic spirochete infections, i.e. Lyme disease).

✦ Origins in training

- A too-rapid increase in the frequency or intensity of training, especially after a period of rest following an injury or foaling.

- Insufficient recovery/cool-down time. A good cool-down should be active, last 20 minutes after work at a sustained pace, and be followed by rest in a quiet, clean place where the horse can relax easily.

- Change of surface (outdoor track, gravel, pavement, sand…).

Fatigue weakens the horse's body until it uses up its own vital energy, which is necessary for healing. Overtraining syndrome causes the horse to lose morale. Plan for cycles of training and rest. Building up an imbalanced horse without correcting his imbalance only reinforces it.

It is best to gain flexibility in an area of the body before building strength or tone. This improves its shock absorption and "bounce," and contributes to making movement more ergonomic. The horse will need less force to perform the same exercise. Direct results include better physical, energetic, emotional, and mental availability of your horse, and prevention of musculotendinous and joint overloads. Stretching prevents or decreases mechanical wear, too.

CHAPTER 3

THE NEUROMUSCULAR STRETCHING METHOD

Principles

The neuromuscular stretching method is broken down into five phases. First, we establish an "inventory" of the different joints. Then, we perform an assessment of the muscle chains involved. The third phase consists—depending on what has been observed and deduced from the preceding tests—of executing a process of gradual tissue release by requesting specific motions and by stretching.

The advantage of this method is that you can carry out passive mobilizations for the horse that he cannot do either alone or mounted.

The horse is mobilized in his most balanced position, starting on all four feet. Each maneuver generates new demands on the sensory receptors (eyes, hooves, vestibular system, spine, cranio-mandibular apparatus, etc.), and the resulting information is analyzed and immediately integrated by the posture control system. The muscular system reacts almost immediately with finesse, strength, and adaptive reflex.

Advice for beginners
Stretching, like any manual technique, must be experienced, felt, and then refined. Only practice and guided analysis of different cases will allow you to work on your conscious sensitivity, assess the sensations of guiding a horse through a stretch, and evolve as a practitioner. The first cases you work through will give you experience that will form the sampling base of perceptions necessary to maximize the effectiveness of the technique and your approach.

Stretching should be thought of as complementary to the horse's usual physical care and sports training, without attempting to replace either.

✦ Phase 1: Find the neutral position of the limb.

The first step is to gently take hold of a limb, offer flexion, and feel the horse's reactions during this request from you. Let's start with a daily observation. When you ask any horse for his foot, he will give it to you more forward, perhaps, or more back, more in or more out. In fact, this position is no accident. You can repeat the request several times as an experiment; any horse will always give you his foot in the same position. This neutral position is shaped by the tensions of the deep muscles of this particular limb. It is the position of least resistance for the limb's joints, which, while in it, are released from the tensions of multi-joint muscles. We then are able to read the defense system of those deeper muscles, which govern postural tone and joint stability. By allowing these tensions to balance, we obtain neutral joint position (which is to say the position that is balanced between the reciprocal tensions of agonist and antagonist muscles). After remaining in this position for ten seconds, it will be the starting point for the stretching movement, the direction of which will be the one indicated to you by the neutral position. This position, in my opinion, is quite useful, and is suitable for practicing all treatments on the limb in question (cleaning the feet, massaging, penetrating ointments or essential oils, etc).

✦ Phase 2: Perform an assessment of the joint.

Passive analytical mobilization involves passively mobilizing a joint from a neutral position (and by "passively" I mean without any muscular effort or contraction by the horse, so no treats or even muscle stimulation that could help achieve the desired movement), and testing all the joints one by one. By evaluating each joint in its degree of freedom or restriction, in the quality of the resulting movement and the level of pain or listlessness, the practitioner performs a complete joint assessment. This specific passive mobilization of each joint does not allow compensation by any above or underlying joints, unlike active mobilizations. Thus, any restriction of mobility or defensive reaction will not escape us, and will be noted on the follow-up sheet. Mobilization by active stimulation of the horse would not give us the information we need here, and is therefore not sought during this portion of the test. During active contractions of the horse's muscles, no control is possible, other than to see (or not see) the horse's compensations. This phase is a sensitive test by which we will evaluate the movement possible in the joint for its quality and quantity; each of these criteria will be compared to that of the limb on the opposite side, and also to an independent standard (which is acquired with experience, depending on the breeds evaluated and the sport practiced by the horses). These criteria can be compared over time for the same horse in order to follow his progress.

In the event of a defensive reaction at the end of a passive movement, it should be noted at what position and intensity this took place and what the type of defensive reaction was. A defensive reaction may come in the form of withdrawal of the mobilized limb, or the transfer of weight in the direction of the movement of the mobilization, thus releasing joint tension. One of the criteria for joint comfort is a sensation of elasticity at the end of the movement.

The range of motion for this joint will be compared with the same joint on the other side, in order to detect any asymmetry between the right and left sides. It is also possible to find you have a feeling of general stiffness coming through more in one of your hands than in the other, during these tests. If most of the joint tests show great flexibility, but some joints have little, this is a sign of stiffening of the osteo-articular system in a specific region, most likely due to a past pathological issue having healed but not without leaving significant traces of fibrosis. Note the behavior of the horse during these tests.

If a joint test is painful, this could be a sign of contraindication for stretching, and an indication to seek veterinary advice. Pain tells the rider not to work his horse, for as long as the pain is present without a veterinary explanation. This little test can prevent excessive work that would lead to more serious injuries.

Quality is a sensitive criterion for assessing how the movement is conducted, and above all for assessing the sensation you get at the end of the movement. The conclusion of a mobilization can fall on a range from soft and elastic to fibrotic, with or without associated pain. It can trigger a defensive movement of the horse, even before you've reached the end of the mobilization.

Quantity will be evaluated as you wish, in degrees or in distance, in relation to a fixed benchmark (the ground, for example). The practitioner will systematically compare the range of motion on each side and note the results on the assessment sheet. There are three possibilities:

- this analytical mobilization does not reveal any problem, which means we can move on to the functional mobilization of muscle chains;

- in case of painless stiffness, the transition to functional mobilization can still be done without too much concern. The compensations for this stiffness that the horse has put in place should be carefully monitored. It is interesting to measure the angles of a joint's range of motion and compare them across sessions;

- in the event of pain or defensive reaction, the priority must be to check with the horse's veterinary care team and discover whether this defense comes from a traumatic, rheumatic, or infected joint problem, or a skin reaction. Unless the veterinarian or the trainer advises otherwise, this joint should not be integrated into the functional mobilization routine.

As you can imagine, these tests are able to detect possible problems early, long before any outward signs of lameness are seen or felt by a rider. Thus, treatment can be carried out quickly, which will prevent lengthy downtimes that slow down competition or training. In the event that the horse's training remains compatible with his medical care, this assessment will make it possible to orient that training to take into account the practical capabilities of the horse. If you have any doubts, it is better to take a break from training and give the horse either full or moderate rest, depending on the clinical assessment. Retest the next day and make your decision afresh. Better to lose a work-out than to do that one session too many that makes the problem worse.

Each test maneuver can be done once or twice. The first sensations are always the best, so trust what you feel.

There is a tendency for beginners to want to guarantee that they've gotten the "correct" results by performing each maneuver at least four or five times. This increases the time it takes to make it through each test, and the horse ends up getting impatient.

✦ Phase 3: Take stock of the state of each muscle chain.

By "muscle chain," I mean all the muscles used to mobilize the limb or the spine in one direction. The retraction of a muscle chain creates muscle and joint compensations in the limb and around the thoracic-vertebral axis. These retractions can be due to pain, the after-effects of trauma, physical deformities, emotional or mental stress, or poor posture. They will only be increased by toning the muscle chain.

By convention, stretching a limb forward causes stretching of its posterior muscle chain; stretching a limb inward, toward the midline, pulls on its outer muscle chain. For the axial muscle chains of the spine, we speak of the ventral chain, comprising all the muscles located under the anteroposterior axis of the horse, and the dorsal chain, made up of all the muscles located above this same axis. Side chains are named for the right or left side.

To reharmonize a joint possessing movement in three dimensions with osteopathy, it is taught that regulating two of the three dimensions is sufficient for the third to release automatically.

This is why we will not be testing the rotational muscle chains. The muscle chains governing two dimensions are enough.

During this test, I find it important to inspect and palpate whichever muscle chain is being stretched (look for signs: a skin lesion, heat in a very localized point, pain on palpation, swelling or hollow suggesting a traumatic injury, etc). This protocol seems amply justified to me if the chain generates a defensive reaction in the horse during its test.

✦ Phase 4: Develop the stretching treatment plan.

Following the tests of the ventral and dorsal chains of the spine, or of the anteroposterior and lateral chains of the limbs, we determine the easiest movement for each limb and spinal area.

Stretching will be done in the direction in which the two chains of the limb move the most easily, or in the direction allowing easy movement of the tested vertebral zone.

✦ Phase 5: Heal by stretching.

For each limb and vertebral axis, stretching will consist of holding the stretching position determined by the muscle tests for 3 minutes.

Passive stretch

After remaining for about ten seconds in the neutral position, the practitioner should then let the limb slowly unfold in the direction indicated by the muscle tests, until a very slight resistance is felt under the fingers.

Then, maintain the limb in this position in a way that is reassuring for the horse, until he lets go. Take a hind limb, for example; the neutral joint position will be in front and toward the midline. You therefore ask the horse to go a little further in his extension in this direction, forwards and inwards.

The very concept of this method is built on the premise that stretching must never be painful. Very quickly, the horse should begin to release, and the practitioner should feel a certain tension melt away in the limb. This hold can last anywhere from 15 to 90 seconds, it doesn't matter—and it is, moreover, the horse who will determine that the exercise is over by retaking control of his limb, either in its original position or while accompanying the stretch and searching for support. Most of the time it's the horse; sometimes the horse falls asleep during the treatment, and it is the practitioner who releases the horse from the stretch. When performing a stretch, it is common for the muscles to start to twitch for a few seconds before relaxing completely. The practitioner then feels a melting of tension, often accompanied by a sigh from the horse. The first few times, it's important to leave the horse with a pleasant feeling. Since this exercise is new to him, he may get impatient, not knowing exactly what to expect from it. Shorten the session now, and in two days, it will be easy for you to stay 3 minutes with the relaxation of your horse. These two times will be repeated two to three times depending on the time and the specific needs of the horse.

The tension in the musculofascial structures generated by this stretching is on the order of a quarter of a pound. It's lower than that generated by the horse's own voluntary dynamic movement, and even less than that generated when the horse rolls over and stands up. There is therefore no risk of damaging the tissues of your horse with the technique described here.

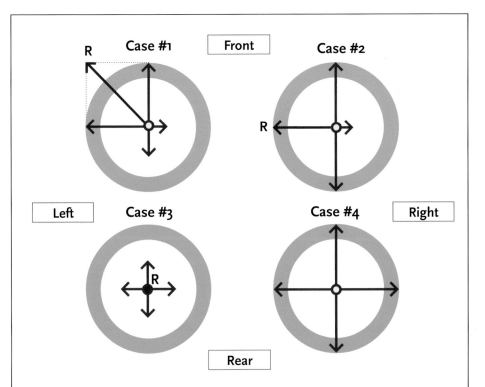

Let's consider some examples and special cases:

- **Case #1:** The direction of greatest ease of movement for the anteroposterior chain is toward the front, and for the lateral chain, it's away from the midline. The result (the arrow labeled R) will be a stretching in front and out (arrow).
- **Case #2:** There is ease of movement for the anteroposterior chain in both directions. No more work is necessary for this muscle chain. There is ease of movement for the side chain when moving toward the midline. The result will be stretching toward the midline.

Two special cases:

- **Case #3:** All the muscle chains are locked; stretching is not indicated. Only the maintenance through quadruple flexion can release the situation, likely within one or two days, by maintaining a bent position of the limb for 3 seconds or more. This case occurs in horses with lower back pain.
- **Case #4:** All the muscle chains are free. With range of motion already being at its best, stretching will then take place more in order to focus and steady the horse before a competition—an emotional effort that will bring him closer to his rider in doing it, more than an effort to achieve muscular regulation.

Variations depending on the objectives

The technique described above is oriented towards in-depth work aiming to rebalance the horse, and refocus him as well as possible.

Stretching can also be used before exercise in training and then in competition.

Muscle stimulation

When the practitioner feels a relaxation of muscle and a realignment of the joints, it's also possible, in the last phase of the stretch, to stretch gently farther in order to stimulate a reaction of contraction in the stretched muscles. The practitioner should slightly oppose the contraction and return of the limb to its original position, in order to guide this return and train the muscle to work in unusual positions. The sensory receptors of the joints and muscles are stimulated and reprogrammed to enhance strength and positional awareness (proprioception) of the corresponding muscle chain.

The true difficulty of learning to perform this technique of equine stretching lies in the need to educate the hands and develop sensitivity. Indeed, you have to set the mind aside and put all your attention into the task of listening to what you are feeling. We are here to listen to the story the horse's tissues have to tell us, and to follow the directions they give us, not to impose on them the narrative we think we should hear or feel. There are endless possibilities; the hands must let themselves follow the sometimes surprising path that the horse's body offers.

When you discover a stubborn muscle chain that gives you the feeling there is no change occurring when you stretch it, then do not push the issue; there are undoubtedly good reasons why this part of the body isn't surrendering its tension. It is preferable to favor the easiest movements for that muscle chain, and keep going.

Often, by working on the opposite limb later, you will release the reluctant side.

Stretching: a way to regulate the energy of the meridians

In traditional Chinese medicine (TCM), the muscles correspond in certain respects with the twelve meridians—the paths through which life energy, qi, flows. Thus, adherents of TCM might reason that there may be a connection between stretching of the tendino muscular meridians and other aspects of TCM, such as the law of the five elements. This association between the neuromuscular physiology of stretching and the conceptualization of life-energy pathways in TCM has yet to be codified for use by TCM practitioners, but the potential is there.

Adaptation of the technique to achieve a chosen goal

Here are some technical variations of the practice of stretching for your horse, depending on the reasons for using the technique.

First variation—maintenance and preventive stretching: Your horse is doing well, and you want to keep him in good health and promote good biomechanics and postural balance, while desensitizing him to unusual movements. This is an ideal practice for young horses. Use of stretching technique will then be aimed at repeating all joint and muscle tests, focusing especially on developing a positive relationship between the horse and the practitioner. Start with short sessions, associated with enjoyable relaxation, then progress to practicing stretching for at least 3 minutes per limb, if necessary. The hula-hoop technique (see p. 102) is particularly suitable as a general technique that desensitizes the horse and gradually eliminates any fear of having his body touched or manipulated.

In order to gradually develop the muscular strength of an athlete without placing too much strain on the musculoskeletal system, a stretching program should be planned. That will guarantee a balanced relationship between strength, flexibility, elasticity, and speed. Therefore, it is a worthwhile daily exercise to be put in place, especially with growing horses, in order to lay a good foundation.

Second variation—curative stretching: Your horse suffers from some kind of chronic pathology. Whether confined in his stall or in rehabilitative care, on the advice of your osteopath and your veterinarian, a stretching and massage program is essential for the proper recovery of your horse. Rebalancing his postural system ensures the mobility condition that was troubling him does not return, and that any compensations caused by training or equipment are dealt with as well. Perform the stretching technique in accordance with the results of the tests (the tests begin on p. 63), which will have to be repeated every three days or so in order to be as precise as possible, depending on the progress of the horse's rehabilitation. When the horse resumes active rehabilitation exercises (the first gallops at a brisk pace, for example), there can be pain associated with the rupture of tissue adhesions often accompanied by edema. This is completely normal, but you have to deal with it as a team with the advice of veterinarians.

Please note: stretching in and of itself should never cause pain. The strength of this stretching technique is that if you stick to it, you can't go wrong, and you protect both your horse and yourself.

Third variation—stretching before and after exertion: Your horse is an athlete, or you go for trail rides, and you want to prepare him for exertion and allow him better recovery in the aftermath of extended exercise.

• Stretching in preparation for exertion: On a physiological level, exertion is associated with the orthosympathetic nervous system, which controls the respiratory, vascular, muscular adaptation systems, etc., in order to maximize efficiency during a "fight or flight" response.

• Warming up increases the heart rate and helps to raise the temperature of muscle tissues, which promotes the sliding of muscle fibers against each other. It dilates vessels, bringing blood, and therefore oxygen, to stressed muscle fibers. It accelerates the speed of nerve conduction, awakens the neuromuscular and neuro-articular receptors, increases the awareness of the proprioceptive regulation system, puts the horse-and-rider pair in a state of psychological preparedness, and promotes sweating (awakening the thermal regulation system and enabling the release of toxins).

Stretching should be included in the warm-up, but does not replace it. Stretching will strengthen the horse's psychological preparedness, allow him to relieve stress and tension, and awaken his body awareness by activating sensory receptors in the joints in unusual positions.

The practitioner explores the physiological range of motion with small joint movements, then goes to the limit of musculo-tendon stretches to alert the nervous system that it must refine its settings. These stimuli at the end of the stretching movement cause the horse to react to the stretched limb, and thus prepare the limb to contract at the end of the stroke. The horse then understands that his body can perform well at the limit of his range of motion. By performing these techniques regularly, you condition the horse to prepare for exertion in the same way that he must be trained to urinate between the first warm-up and the start of a work session. How can he possibly release all physical tension if his bladder is full?

The stretching session in this case will be short (one minute per limb or per vertebral zone) and invigorating. If your horse is nervous, start the same procedure and then, while on the way to enter the work area, do the tongue stretch—you can even continue it until you have reached the work area.

Exercise recovery stretching: on a physiological level, recovery from a period of exercise is associated with the parasympathetic nervous system, which organizes the respiratory, vascular, and muscular adaptation systems, and more, in order to maximize efficiency during recovery, wound healing, digestion, and procreation.

Muscle contraction is the result of a electro-biochemical reaction that generates toxins (lactic acids, in particular, during anaerobic work without oxygen), which is to say wastes that must be transformed or eliminated by the body.

As a result of these toxins and wastes accumulating, the muscle becomes tense, the range of motion is reduced, and sometimes pain appears, resulting in lameness. In the days following, there are aches and contractures, with fetlocks or hocks thickened by poor circulation. The spasmed muscles constrict the veins and lymphatic system, which then have great difficulty circulating fluid. The resulting swelling can compress nerves and cause radiating pain throughout the area served by the affected nerves (sciatica).

The condition of a horse's muscles after exertion depends on his level of training and the work that has been asked of him. Overworked muscle tends to shorten and fill up with toxins; the feeling of fatigue weighs on the horse, and certain muscle groups are intermittently painful.

A stretching session should be carried out only after having completed an active recovery period of 10 to 15 minutes of gallop or trot, at approximately 60% of the level of effort expended during the work session—this will constitute aerobic work, which allows the blood vessels within the muscles to remain sufficiently dilated to maintain blood flow and oxygen supply, and carry away waste accumulated during work, allowing the muscles to recharge their batteries. A good hot rinse-off (except on inflammatory areas) is another tool to keep the superficial vessels dilated; then dry the horse off.

The tensions in the horse after exertion are proportional to the compensatory forces that allowed him to carry out his work (see chapter 2). It is often very interesting to compare the horse's range of motion before and after a work session. Stretching in the recovery phase serves as a post-exertion assessment, and makes it possible to determine, through the reactions of the horse, the areas to be monitored, cooled, heated, massaged, or, if you are concerned, shown to the veterinarian for an examination and differential diagnosis.

A recovery-phase stretching session should be long (3 minutes per limb), and possibly preceded by the hula-hoop technique (see p. 102) if the horse is really tense, focused towards light stretching without requiring muscle contraction. The horse must be brought to a state of calm. He can eat his hay during the session, and very often you'll find he has a tendency to doze off.

Session setup and procedure

✦ Warm up the horse

It is a good idea to walk the horse in hand a few minutes before undertaking a session. This will allow him to rebalance his tensions to some degree when he comes out of his stall, and rouses him out of any drowsiness. Gentle movement increases circulation and the visco-elasticity of connective tissues, by generating a slight rise in internal temperature. Observing the first "cold" steps at the start of a warm-up gives good information on the condition of the horse. Oftentimes, he will take the opportunity to stretch naturally. Assess the meaning of the stretches he offers on his own, and the area of his body that is involved; you will almost certainly find this information repeated when you are assessing the responses of his tissues during the stretches later. This is his way of indicating his needs to anyone who knows how to look at him.

✦ Approaching the horse
Location

You have to choose a quiet, comfortable place, preferably one that is familiar to the horse and will allow him to relax. It can be in his stall on straw or shavings, in the grooming area, or in the arena on sand. It is absolutely imperative to avoid an uneven or sloping surface, which would alter the horse's balance and trigger reflexive compensatory contractures.

The horse should be able to stand square, and the practitioner should have enough space to move around the horse without any risk of ending up trapped against a wall or any object that could injure either of them.

Interaction

Talk to the horse in a friendly manner, avoiding any sudden gestures, in order to give him confidence, especially when you are behind him.

Even when fully trained and docile, the horse can, with an abrupt movement, hurt you. Usually it is fear that makes him dangerous. Give him time to get used to your presence and then to your approach. The relationship established between you and him must be based on trust and listening, and any sense that you should hold power over him must be banished.

Assistance

For safety reasons, during the first few sessions, a third person should hold the horse by the halter or a lead rope, always standing *on the same side as the practitioner* when the practitioner is working on the back or hindquarters. Thus, if there is a reaction, the horse will free himself by moving away from them both, and will not endanger either human.

Avoid having a session just before the horse's mealtime, or passing fillies under the nose of a stallion that you are stretching, and rule out any other distracting event that might excite the horse.

✦ When to practice stretching

As we will see in chapter 4, stretching is useful when warming up, recovering from exertion, and as part of a flexibility training program.

As noted previously, warming up increases the heart rate, and helps raise the temperature of the muscle tissue, which promotes the sliding of muscle fibers, ligaments, and fasciae against each other. Warming up also dilates the blood vessels to increase

Safety tips:

- Protect your back.
- Protect your feet with good shoes.
- Wear gloves, which will protect you against cold or risk of injury from the edges of horseshoes.
- Dress comfortably.
- Work in a quiet place.
- Be calm and attentive about everything you are doing.
- Make sure you can move all the way around the horse safely.
- Place the horse's head at the rear of his stall, if that's where you're working, so he can't be distracted by anything visible through the stall door.
- Have the horse guided by an assistant, who is always standing on the same side of the space as you are.
- Record notes and observations of your horse during the session on a piece of paper or in a notebook you can refer to later.
- Never force a stretch.

circulation, and therefore deliver more oxygen, to stressed muscle fibers. It accelerates the speed of nerve conduction, puts the horse-and-rider pair in a state of psychological readiness, and promotes sweating (a system of thermal regulation that enables the release of toxins).

Stretching should be included in the warm-up phase, but cannot replace it. A stretching session will strengthen the psychological preparedness of the horse, allow him to release the tensions of stress, and will awaken his body awareness by triggering information from the joint receptors in unusual positions.

Recovery from exertion

As previously explained, muscle contraction is the result of a electro-biochemical reaction that generates toxins (lactic acids, in particular, during anaerobic work without oxygen), which is to say wastes that must be transformed or eliminated by the body.

The muscles becomes tense, range of motion is reduced, and sometimes pain appears, resulting in lameness. In the days that follow, there are aches and contractures with edema in the fetlocks or hocks, due to poor outgoing circulation (the spasmed muscles constrict veins and lymphatic vessels which pass through fascia, and therefore outgoing drainage of waste from the muscle cells is reduced or impossible).

The best recovery session is an active recovery session. 5 to 10 minutes after the main work session, stress-free exercise should resume for 10 to 20 minutes at an easy pace for the horse—a slow canter or an easy trot—at a level around 60% of what was

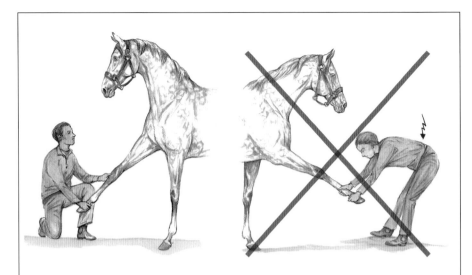

The position of the practitioner is essential. It's about mobilizing the horse through firm, gentle, steady holds. Considering the horse weighs as much as he does, you must avoid straining your back in your efforts to free his! I advise you to warm up at the same time as the horse and then, during the session, to always make sure to bend at the knees and keep your spine as straight as possible. Use your weight rather than your strength, and make the direction of pull as close to your center of gravity as possible, between the belly button and the hips.

asked of him during the main work session. By reducing the degree of effort required and the amount of stress on the body, it will be possible for the muscles to oxygenate and drain. This kind of aerobic work (work light enough to permit oxygen flow) generates waste products that are immediately drained away by the body, and is very useful for recovering from anaerobic work.

A good rinse-off should then be followed by a stretching session.

The condition of a horse's muscles after exertion depends on his level of training and the work that has been asked of him. Overworked muscle tends to shorten and fill up with toxins; the feeling of fatigue weighs on the horse, and certain muscle groups are intermittently painful.

This kind of stretching session should be focused around light stretches that do not require any active contraction on the part of the horse. Let us remember that the tensions in the horse after exertion are proportional to the compensatory forces that allowed him to carry out his work (see chapter 2). It is often very interesting to compare the horse's range of motion before and after a work session, and this will let you determine the areas to be monitored, cooled, heated, or massaged.

A flexibility training program

In order to gradually develop the muscular strength of an athlete without placing too much strain on the musculoskeletal system, a stretching program should be planned. One that will guarantee a balanced relationship between strength, flexibility, elasticity, and speed. It's a worthwhile daily exercise to be put in place, especially with growing horses, in order to lay a good foundation.

✦ Where to begin

In the event of existing pathology, equine health professionals will show you exactly what they want you to do in the best interests of the horse's rehabilitation.

When there is no acute pathology, as part of preventative care for the neuro-musculoskeletal system, there is no mandatory starting place: you are free to begin the session with the head, back, forelegs, or hindquarters. Experience shows that it is better to start as far as possible from a potential problem.

Once connection and feel have been established, to me it seems worthwhilie to always respect that, so that the horse is able to fully release his tension without hesitation. The first few sessions must be carried out with special attention to ensure that they are good experiences for the horse. Stretching should not hurt or cause too sudden a reaction; this is what guarantees an increase in muscle flexibility and range of motion.

Gain in range of motion through stretching is based on the quality of your (slow, gentle) resistance to the contraction of the muscles when the horse reaches the limit of the stretch and pulls back, not the strength of the stretch itself.

The comparison of range of motion, degree of muscular release, and quality of joint freedom between the horse's left and right sides will allow you to better understand the discomforts and potential compensations of the horse, as well as his capabilities during work under saddle.

A stretching session should make it possible to understand the way in which the horse behaves during work sessions. This biomechanical analysis tests the horse's range of motion joint by joint. If, analytically, the horse cannot achieve an appropriate range of motion, he will have functional difficulties and seek to compensate with other joints, which will then be overworked. Asymmetry in muscle size, when one side of the horse is compared to the other, will tell us that these compensations are not recent developments.

✦ Duration and frequency of sessions
Duration

The duration of a stretching session will vary according to the objectives we set for a specific horse, the time available for the session, and, for competition horses, the stage of the horse's preparation. The type of session will differ depending on whether it is a warm-up, a recovery period between two work sessions, a cool-down at the end of a work session, or a specific effort for the purpose of "unlocking" a restricted area.

Carrying out a complete session on a horse familiar with this stretching method should take about 10 minutes. The first few times, though, it should take between 20 and 30 minutes. A new way of thinking about your warm-up would be to incorporate these 10 minutes of stretching without increasing the warm-up's total duration. For show horses, this means slightly reducing the amount of time to relax in the walk and trot, starting the stretching session, and then proceeding to the starting area.

For trotters, a stretching session seems to be best positioned during the warm-up heat of a race, reducing the time spent walking. For some horses, we can replace a warm-up heat with stretching and work our way through a "true" warm-up just before the last heat of the race begins.

Frequency

Repeating stretching sessions daily is part of this stretching technique. I recommend it very often after an osteopathic treatment. After a treatment, the horse finds himself with a new and expanded range of motion, but he has not yet integrated it into his way of moving, and he will not use that expanded ability until he has assimilated it. In this context, stretching can be thought of as a kind of sensory (proprioceptive) rehabilitation, aimed at integrating the horse's improved range of movement with his subconscious body awareness. It is also, for the rider or the trainer who will perform these sessions, an opportunity to follow the progress of the horse and to understand what it will be possible to ask of the horse once mounted.

✦ The reactions of the horse following a session

The internal adjustments made by a passive stretching session can, like any harmonizing treatment, create a feeling of general relaxation. The horse sometimes lets himself go to sleep.

If we stimulate muscle contractions, there will be harmonization and resolution of tension, while at the same time maintaining a muscle tone and energy level suitable for work.

Precautions

As we have seen, stretching is based on stimulating self-regulation. It can cause powerful toxin purges during the first three sessions. As a rule, the horse feels tired, and he is calm. By the next day, he may be stiffer, re-finding his balance following the new information about his body that the session gave him. If the horse is used to going to the paddock, let him go. Just remember to be careful with him, even if you are working him, as he may taken by surprise by the change in his range of motion.

When stretching a horse that has never been stretched, or hasn't been stretched for a long time, it is wise to start with short sessions. The message conveyed to the horse should, above all, make him understand the playful, pleasant, soothing nature of this "new game." This will also help to eliminate overly strong reactions the next day.

It would be a mistake to start using this technique within three days of an important competition.

As if it were the first time! Listen to, feel, and ride your mount differently.

What to do after a session

The rider must start fresh with her horse, listening to what her mount can tell her, in a different place than she was before the treatment.

For example: in show jumping, with certain difficult horses, riders sometimes tend to use artificial aids in order to try to find a solution. They lengthen their spurs, or use the whip more often and more forcefully.

These old habits should be set aside. It will be necessary to begin anew, with the horse free of any of these added constraints, as if it were the first time. Avoid using a forceful bit, excessive spurs, or too-strong reins.

✦ The limits of stretching

Setting aside the contraindications already mentioned, the effectiveness of stretching sessions will be visible day by day. When you no longer notice improvement, your horse has reached the peak benefit he is currently able to derive from stretching. That is the time to refocus your efforts on maintenance sessions, depending on the horse's work and sporting level.

If, despite the general gains in range of motion, signs of stiffness or discomfort persist, it is time to bring in a professional from your horse's healthcare team, whose examination you can easily steer in the right direction thanks to your joint tests.

If a particularly tight area shows no progress despite work spanning the entire body, it's time to review all the points capable of showing signs of dysfunction (see chapter 1).

In fact, by using the limbs to work the spine, we will respect the physiology of the joints. Let the professionals take direct action on the vertebrae.

If no change in a problem is noted after six or seven days, with one or two daily stretching sessions, a veterinarian should be consulted in order to establish a diagnosis. There are problems for which stretching can do nothing (except help to release all compensations for the problem, and not the problem itself). This is where the limits of stretching lie.

In summary

After testing various joints and muscle chains, the horse should be offered a stretch in the area where it is most comfortable. As the stretch is released, we can mobilize the stiffer areas.

There are two ways of practicing stretching:
* passive stretching, held for a long time without asking for a reaction at the end of the stretch;
* passive stretching, held and ending with a request for the horse to react with a movement that contracts the muscle.

The first corresponds more to a posture held for quite a while, and will be used in recovery after exertion and in programs aimed at improving range of motion.

The second will be used as a way to awaken body awareness, as a warm-up, or between two work sessions because it stimulates muscle chains and increases postural tone.

These two methods can be supplemented by active stretching, in particular on the level of the spine (see chapter 7, p. 100).

CHAPTER 4

INDICATIONS AND CONTRAINDICATIONS FOR STRETCHING

Indications

The indications for stretching fall into four categories.

✦ Mechanical action

By its mechanical action, stretching:

* allows you to lengthen the muscles, increase range of motion in stride, and release tension from the back blocked by muscles that are too short. It facilitates engagement in your horse, and makes exercises doable when they were previously impossible to perform;

* maintains flexibility, through prolonging specific joint postures. Stretching is particularly useful in the aftermath of physical trauma, to recover harmony of movement and release adhesions from scar tissue;

* promotes good recovery after exercise by lengthening muscle fibers, which tend to remain shortened following exertion otherwise;

* contributes to better breathing by releasing all chest tension. The diaphragm relaxes and the horse recovers bounce and fluidity of movement;

* maintains good blood circulation, responsible for oxygenation, nutrition, and tissue drainage. Thus, the tissues are more resistant to damage and repair themselves faster.

✦ Development of the relationship between horse and human

On a relational and emotional level, stretching:

- allows the horse to be taught respect for everyone. In young horses, stretching is a wonderful tool to prepare for other kinds of handling;

- contributes to the education of the rider in understanding her partner. The very act of taking time to stretch the horse sensitizes the rider to the progress of her mount, which means she will be better able to appreciate the amount of effort she can reasonably ask;

- helps the rider and the trainer orient their work in a more personalized and efficient way, thanks to an improved understanding of the functioning of the horse, on both psychological and biomechanical levels.

✦ Information transmitted to the nervous system

Through the information transmitted to the nervous system, stretching allows:

- relaxation of muscle chains due to prolonged stretching postures, which stimulate internal sensory receptors. The brain is then able to cue the body to relax;

- improved coordination of the horse and his perception of his body in space, which is invaluable in training;

- toning of a stretched muscle in its longest position. This gives it more resistance to the type of stress created by exertion;

- reprogramming of the muscular and ligamentary systems by increasing movement speed and improving reflexes controlling movement during exertion. This reprogramming is even more necessary in the event of trauma to the tissues;

- deep relaxation of the muscles and release of nervous tension, while at the same time improving the reaction speed of the muscles;

- warming up in preparation for exertion, to prepare the brain and focus the horse's attention on upcoming activities. The postural tone is put on alert.

✦ Preventive action

Used preventively, stretching allows:

- tests of the condition of muscles and joints, and helps to differentiate a muscle problem from a joint problem;

- evaluation and understanding of each horse according to his constitution, his conformation (long-limbed or short and powerful), and his behavior toward his human partner, eliminating the need for trial-and-error;

- reduction in the risk of injury to muscles, joints, or tendons, by encouraging relaxation, vascularization, and programming of reflexes;

- alleviation of compensatory tension in muscles and joints. This will result in better rest, and the possibility of resuming training without the same problem reoccurring and without adding new levels of compensation that would end up causing new problems;

- prevention of functional degeneration (osteoarthritis, arthritis) appearing with age and depending on the working conditions of the horse;

- reduction in the use of corticosteroids or other non-steroidal anti-inflammatory drugs, which accelerate wear and tear on cartilage during prolonged treatments;

- improvement of the horse's shock-absorbing capacity by "de-rusting" the skeletal structure and re-harmonizing or releasing various muscle tensions;

- reduction in the cost of care required to deal with these many problems.

Contraindications

There are also some contraindications for stretching. Stretching should be avoided:
- if you observe any acute inflammation, trauma, or infection;

- within 48 hours of a severe trauma (risk of hematoma);

- if the horse is experiencing any sharp pain;

- if you observe dangerous behavior in the horse which would put your safety at risk.

If in doubt, do not hesitate to ask your veterinarian.

CHAPTER 5

JOINT
ARTICULATION TESTS

Passive analytical joint mobilization

In a mechanical sense, testing a joint requires locating it anatomically, and clearly determining the two bones to be mobilized and the direction in which to mobilize by focusing on the axis on which you intend to stretch the joint. It is necessary to move slowly and gently from the neutral joint position toward the end of the joint's range of motion, and observe the extent and quality of the movement.

The positioning of the different grips for each hand, as well as the positioning of the feet and the body, is essential. Your stability and peace of mind, as well as your visualization of the movement of the joint, will allow you to obtain optimum relaxation and cooperation from the horse.

Passive analytical joint mobilization consists of mobilizing and testing all the joints one by one, in order to assess their degree of freedom or restriction. This specific mobilization of each joint does not allow for any compensation by other joints. Thus, any restriction of mobility, or defensive reaction, cannot escape us and will be noted on our observation sheet. This portion of the stretching session is a sensory test through which we will be able to assess the degree of movement by its quality and quantity. The horse's two sides will be compared with each other and against an abstract standard (which is learned with experience).

Let's consider an example: when you flex a joint, you stretch its extensor muscles. Visualizing the axis of motion is important to allow you to understand which muscles are being worked, even if you do not know their names. Each joint is thought of as

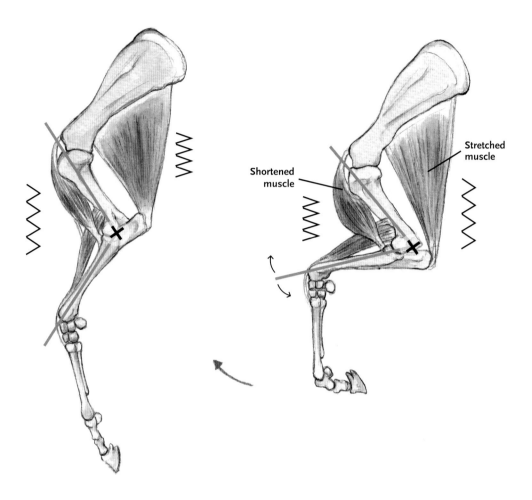

Stretched muscle

Shortened muscle

rotating around an axis; the direction we designate "forward" from this axis is the direction of movement, and, using this definition, it is the muscles behind the axis that will be stretched by the movement, while the muscles in front will be shortened.

The practitioner must take care not to strain her own back with all these tests, by seeking the best possible position. Your postures and grip should be adapted according to your size and strength. The options I offer in this guide are not exhaustive.

Each test maneuver can be done once or twice. The first reactions are always the best, so have confidence in what you feel.

✦ The names of the movements
Movements for limbs

- The movement that brings the two bone segments that form a joint together is called flexion.

- The movement that separates these two bone segments is called extension.

- Movement that brings the lower bone segment closer to the midline of the body is adduction.

- Movement that directs this segment away from the midline is abduction.

- Rotation of a bone that is directed toward the inside of the body is called internal rotation.

- Rotation of a bone that is directed outward is called external rotation.

Movements for the vertebrae

- Movement that inclines the base of one vertebra toward the base of another is called flexion (e.g, the head-down and raised-back position called "roundness").

- Movement that brings the tops of the vertebrae toward each other is called extension (e.g, head in the air or hollow back).

- Lateral tilts allow the horse's body to curve; these movements are more or less equivalent to rotations in limbs.

The limbs

The mobility of the horse's limbs is mainly in the front-to-back direction, i.e. flexion/extension. Only the hips and shoulders are able to explore all three spatial dimensions through movements of rotation and laterality (abduction: outward and adduction: inward). Rotational tests of lower joints can only be performed if they are placed in flexion. On any of the horse's limbs, the uppermost joints are surrounded by a large muscle mass. The lower joints (fetlocks, hocks, and knees), for their part, are stabilized only by nearby tendons and strong ligament attachments. If the horse is standing square at the halt on his four limbs, without going into a supportive posture to relieve weight in any leg, this should be considered evidence that the extension of the lower joints (up to the elbow and stifle) is reasonably good and not painful to the horse. Therefore, we need only test them in flexion. These joints bear over two hundred pounds apiece, at a minimum, in this position at the halt in extension. We would be hard-pressed to manually simulate any stretch in extension as strong as that.

— STRETCH EXERCISES FOR HORSES

✦ Ensuring your safety

Photograph 1: When it comes to joint tests of the hind legs, I offer you this safety grip to grasp the hind leg whose joints you are intending to mobilize. In this photograph, the right hand grasps the foot with the palm against the hoof, and the fingers come to rest on the sole. The left hand can be set across the back of the right to strengthen your grip if the horse is heavy or "restless." Obviously, these tests should only be done if the horse has shown you that he is well behaved and that he respects you. This grip will keep your hand in contact with the horse's foot at all times during mobilizations.

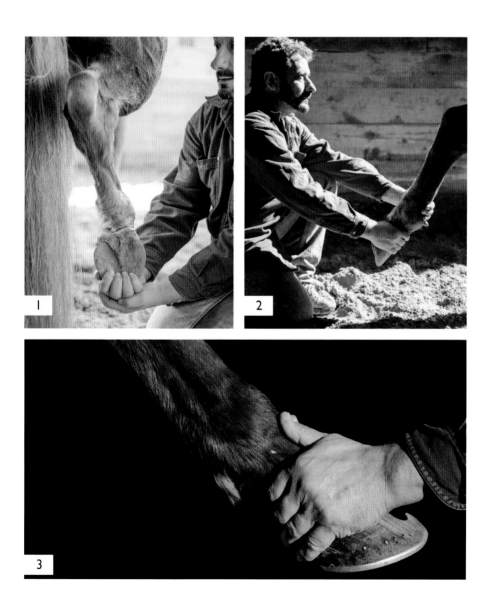

Photograph 2: Here is a safety hold for movements that ask the limbs to go backwards. One hand grasps the pastern. The fingers curve over the anterior surface of the leg (i.e., the side of the leg closer to the horse's face) and the thumb wraps around in opposition—not gripping heavily, but ready to do so if necessary. The other hand grasps the cannon bone, again with the thumb in opposition.

When taking a lowered position, the practitioner should place one knee on the ground. This position is comfortable for performing stretching tests and treatments. If you have to get up quickly for one reason or another, you won't be impeded: the hand gripping the cannon bone, and the rest of you by extension, will automatically be lifted partway because that is the direction in which the horse will first retract his limb.

Photograph 3: Here is a safety hold for movements that ask the limbs to go forward. Both hands grasp the back of the pastern, and the thumbs are placed on its anterior surface. Be careful not to put your fingers under the sole of the foot. Some techniques require being as close to the ground as possible, and sometimes the horse feels unsteady and reflexively tries to seek greater support by setting his hoof down. This grip will prevent any fear or accident.

✦ The forelegs and anterior spine

The anterior part of the thoracic skeleton is held in place by the two shoulder blades. Muscle strength and the balancing of muscle tension makes this shoulder girdle stable. The forelegs support 60-65% of the horse's body weight, as his center of gravity is located closer to the forelegs than the hindquarters. The forelegs have great joint mobility.

Interphalangeal mobilization

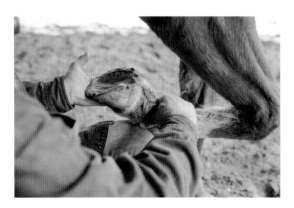

▶ FLEXION-EXTENSION
Bend the knee 90° and grasp the pastern with your right hand, just under the fetlock. The left hand mobilizes with an up-and-down movement of the hoof.

JOINTS OF THE FORELEGS AND ANTERIOR SPINE

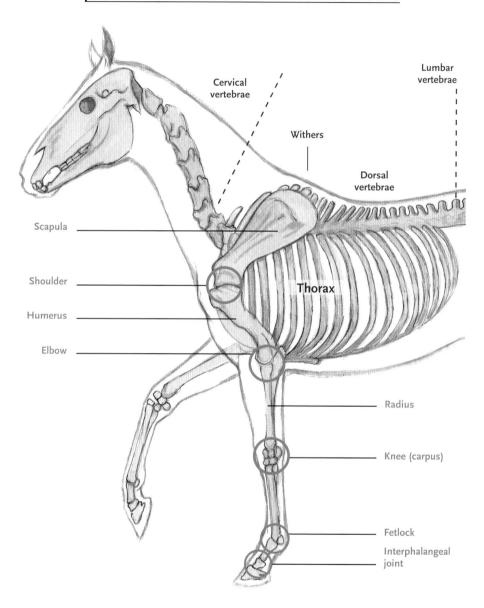

Cervical
vertebrae

Lumbar
vertebrae

Withers

Dorsal
vertebrae

Scapula

Shoulder

Thorax

Humerus

Elbow

Radius

Knee (carpus)

Fetlock

Interphalangeal
joint

SHOULDER GIRDLE

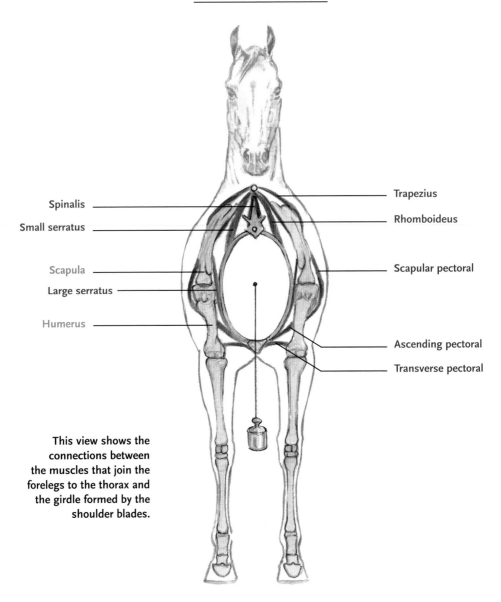

Spinalis

Small serratus

Scapula

Large serratus

Humerus

Trapezius

Rhomboideus

Scapular pectoral

Ascending pectoral

Transverse pectoral

This view shows the connections between the muscles that join the forelegs to the thorax and the girdle formed by the shoulder blades.

Mobilization of the fetlock

The pastern forms a joint with the first phalange and two posterior bones called the sesamoids. Passive mobilization towards extension cannot reach the maximum range of motion for this joint. This is because the ligaments are extremely strong, and already stretch constantly to support the weight of the horse; do not even consider attempting to go further.

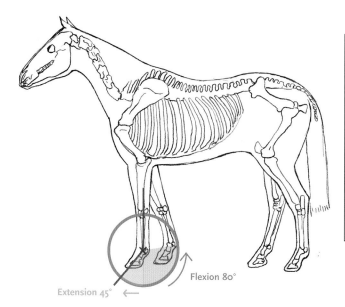

Joint tests are presented from the periphery to the center. The direction of movement and the amplitude of the joint tested are represented by two arrows (blue and green). The axis of movement is in red.

Flexion 80°

Extension 45°

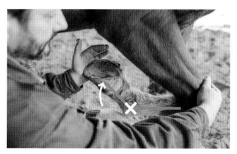

▼ FLEXION-EXTENSION

Bend the knee so that the cannon bone is horizontal, and hold the knee with your right hand. The left hand mobilizes the interphalangeal joints and the fetlock through compressive flexion of the hoof. It is important to increase this stretch until you feel a distinct end-of-motion "stopper" in the fetlock in flexion. In the event of a fetlock problem, this flexion stretch will be positive and will strengthen the fetlock.

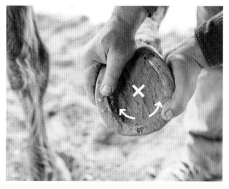

▼ ROTATION

Starting in the neutral position, grasp the hoof with both hands. Internal rotation directs the front of the hoof toward the midline of the horse, and external rotation, away from the horse. Then, with the thumbs, mobilize the sesamoid bones (behind the fetlock).

Knee (carpus) mobilization

While this joint in the foreleg is commonly referred to as the knee, it actually corresponds to the human wrist. The radius and third metacarpal are separated by two rows of small bones.

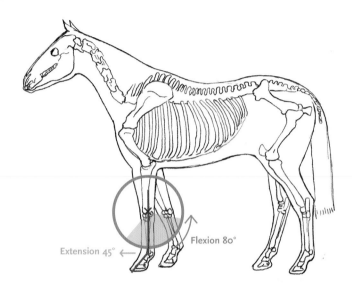

Extension 45° ←

Flexion 80°

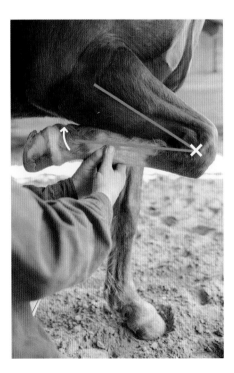

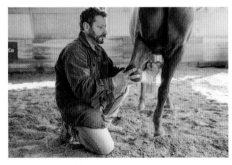

▼ ROTATION-LATERALITY

Grasp the hoof with your left hand, with the right hand placed on the knee. Bend the knee 120°. The right hand pushes sideways, and the other hand keeps the knee oriented on its initial axis. The movement stops when the tip of the elbow moves outward.

▶ FLEXION-EXTENSION

With both hands under the cannon bone, gently lift it to bring it into contact with the radius, letting the carpus (knee) move forward and up (be careful not to hold the foot, as this will cause the rear part of the horse's shoe to bump his elbow).

Elbow mobilization

The elbow connects the humerus to the radius and ulna.

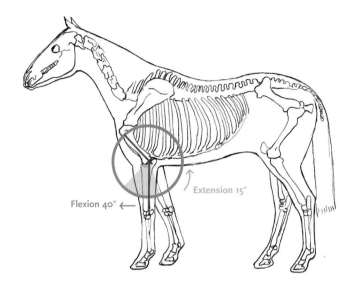

Extension 15°

Flexion 40°

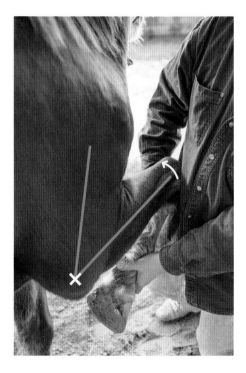

▶ FLEXION

The right hand grasps the back of the foreleg, and the left hand grips the fetlock. Gently lift the carpus (knee), with your right hand moving towards the point of the shoulder to close the angle between the humerus and the radius.

Shoulder mobilization

The shoulder is the most mobile joint in the horse's body. It is made up of the joint between the humerus and the scapula, and the joint formed by the sliding of the scapula over the ribs. It helps orient the horse in all three spatial dimensions.

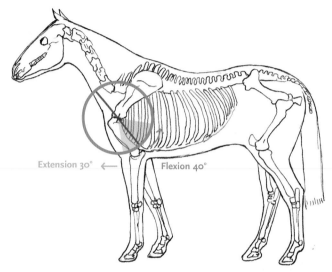

Extension 30° ←   Flexion 40°

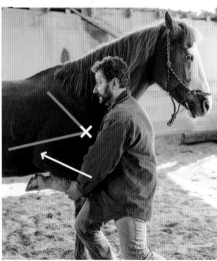

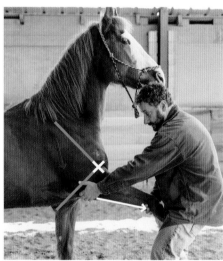

▼ FLEXION

Place the knee of the horse on your thigh, with your right hand under the radius and your left hand supporting the fetlock. Use your body weight as you push towards the horse so that the tip of his elbow points back and up. At the end of this movement, you will see flexion of the upper dorsal vertebrae with elevation of the withers.

▼ EXTENSION

Facing the shoulder, grasp the back of the knee with both hands and gradually lift the front towards you. Depending on the degree of muscle tension, the foot may extend between your thighs. At the end of the movement, you can pull the tip of the elbow forward with your left hand to feel the fully opened angle between the scapula and the humerus.

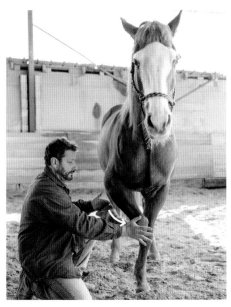

▼ INTERNAL ROTATION

Grasp the hoof with your left hand and hold the cannon bone horizontal, with the knee in your right hand. From this position, push down and in with your right hand and gently pull up and out with your other hand.

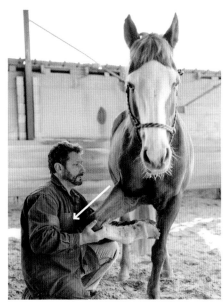

▼ EXTERNAL ROTATION

Use the same grip as for internal rotation. Push with the left hand and gently pull towards you with the right hand.

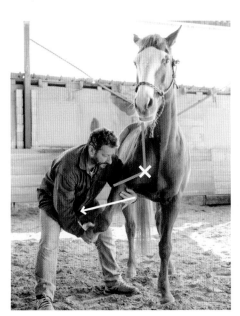

▼ ABDUCTION

Place your left elbow above the horse's elbow. Your right hand should hold the fetlock and maintain a knee flexion angle of about 90°; then use both hands to spread the shoulder apart, pulling out and up.

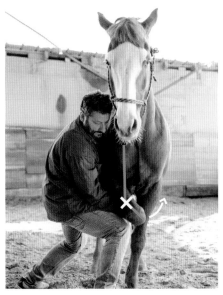

▼ ADDUCTION

Grasp the foot with your left hand and the cannon bone with your right hand. Place your forearm on your thigh, and shift your body weight in and out in order to mobilize the shoulder in adduction.

✦ The hind joints

The hind legs attach to the spine via the pelvic girdle. The iliac bone articulates with the spine through the sacrum and hip bone of the hind leg. Thanks to their biomechanical structure, the hind legs stabilize the horse and provide the bulk of his locomotion. They support 40% of his body weight.

POSTERIOR ARTICULATIONS

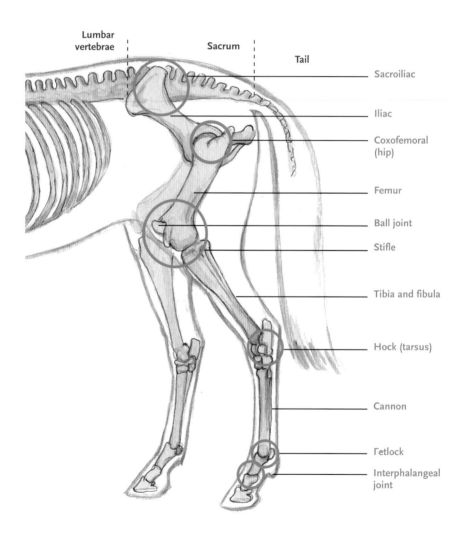

Lumbar vertebrae

Sacrum

Tail

Sacroiliac

Iliac

Coxofemoral (hip)

Femur

Ball joint

Stifle

Tibia and fibula

Hock (tarsus)

Cannon

Fetlock

Interphalangeal joint

Interphalangeal mobilization

The last of the phalanges are tested in both flexion and extension. This mobilization will stretch muscles and ligaments, including the suspensory. It's a great way to stimulate vascular drainage in the foot.

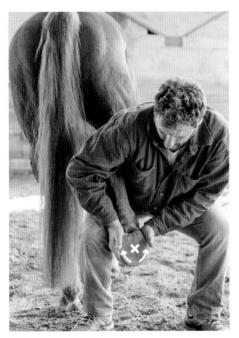 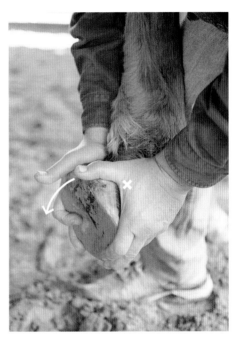

▼ EXTENSION/FLEXION

After grasping the leg, place the fold of the hock on your hip (a "farrier's grip") and find a position of balanced tension between you and the horse. This grip will allow you to effortlessly mobilize the joints with both hands. To protect your back, rest your elbows on your thighs. Use your thumbs to push the bulbs (the rounded areas to either side of the cleft in the frog) down, and your fingers to hook the front edge of the hoof for an extension movement.

Mobilization of the fetlock

The third metatarsus articulates with the first phalange and two posterior bones called the sesamoids. Passive mobilization towards extension cannot reach the maximum range of motion for this joint. This is because the ligaments are extremely strong, and already stretch constantly to support the weight of the horse; do not even consider attempting to go further.

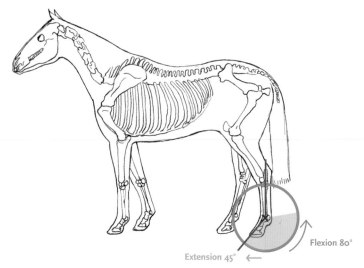

Flexion 80°

Extension 45° ←

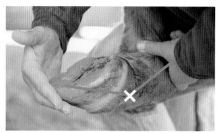

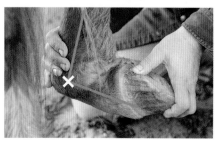

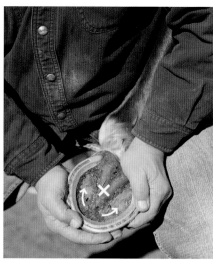

▼ FLEXION

Upper photo: Begin with the same basic grip as on page 67. Your knee supports the cannon bone, and one or both hands move the fetlock into flexion by manipulating the tip of the foot. Lower photo: Variant option, if farrier position proves impossible.

▼ ROTATION

Begin with the same basic grip as for flexion. Your hands grasp the hoof, and rotate on an imaginary longitudinal axis passing through the center of the sole. These rotations involve the interphalangeal joint and the fetlock. Then, with the thumbs, mobilize the sesamoid bones (behind the fetlock).

Mobilization of the hock

The tarsus is a cluster of several rows of bones. It articulates between the tibia and the metatarsus. The hock is surrounded by tendons, which are themselves surrounded by circular fasciae that keep them sliding during movement.

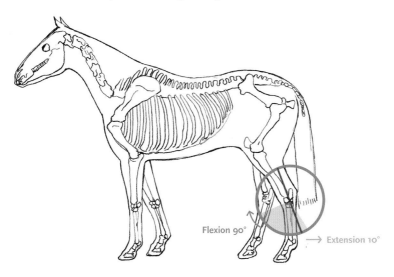

Flexion 90°   → Extension 10°

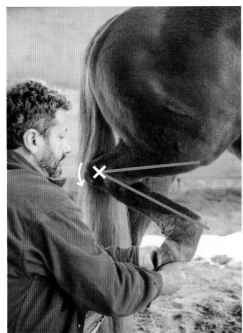

▼ FLEXION

Grasp the hoof securely with your hands. Bend the hind leg to bring the fetlock closer to the knee, while leaving the stifle unconstrained.

Stifle mobilization

This joint corresponds to the knee in humans. It brings together the femur, the tibia, and the patella. It is a very elaborate joint because it must be very mobile in flexion, but stable under pressure. The main movement of the stifle is flexion-extension. The stifle locks when in extension, and allows minimal rotations when in flexion.

Rotational movements can only be done by flexing the stifle in order to relax the collateral ligaments. To check the movement of the rotating femur, just watch the anterior tuberosity of the tibia move during the test.

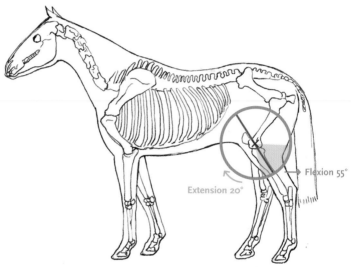

Flexion 55°

Extension 20°

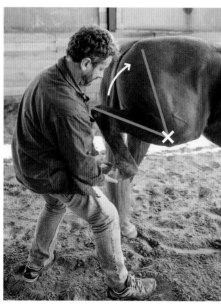

▼ FLEXION
Grasp the hoof securely with your hands. Bend the hind leg to bring the point of the hock as close as possible to the point of the buttock.

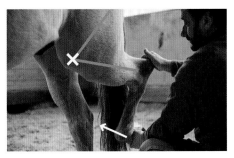

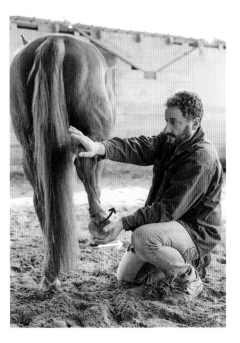

INTERNAL ROTATION ▼

Your right hand grasps the point of the hock, and your left hand grips the leg by the hoof or pastern. Rest your left wrist on your knee. The cannon bone must be vertical, and the hock must be flexed at 90°. You anchor a fixed point with your right hand, and your left hand pushes the foot away from you to create internal rotation in the stifle.

EXTERNAL ROTATION ◄

Use the same grip as for internal rotation, but this time your left hand pulls the foot toward you to create external rotation in the stifle.

Hip mobilization

The hip connects the posterior to the pelvic girdle. Its function is to orient the limb in all directions, while having a role of stability. The interlocking of the head of the femur in the pelvis gives it stability and allows it to withstand significant forces. It is surrounded by very powerful ligaments, as well as an impressive mass of muscles.

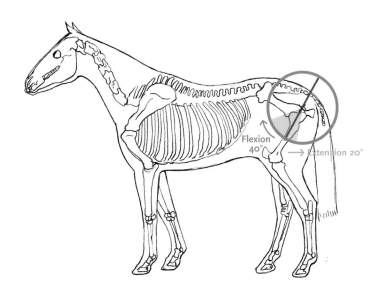

Flexion 40°

Extension 20°

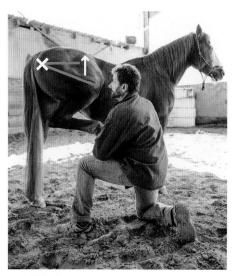

▼ FLEXION

Grasp the hoof with your hands. Bend the hind leg to bring the stifle forward and upward. The hind leg will be folded like an accordion. Depending on the size of the horse, you will need to kneel high, or even stand, until you feel the stretch caused by the tilt of the pelvis reach a natural limit.

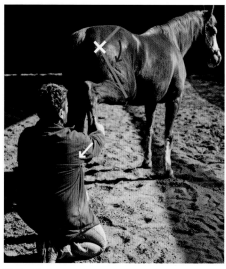

▼ EXTENSION

Grasp the cannon bone with your right hand, with the thumb in opposition but not digging in (safety grip). With your left hand, grab the pastern. Gradually draw the hind leg backward.

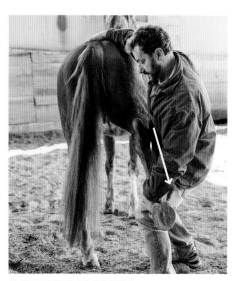

▼ EXTENSION (VARIATION)

Grasp the fetlock with your left hand, and gradually draw the hind leg backward to rest it on your left knee. Let the horse relax. Your right hand can relax the horse's muscles with a reassuring touch, and balance you at the same time. Place most of your body weight on your right foot, to avoid too much compression on the foot on which the weight of horse's cannon bone is already resting.

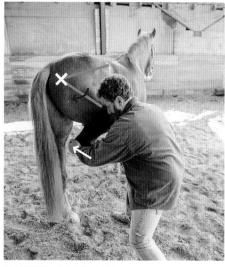

▼ EXTERNAL ROTATION

Grasp the point of the hock with your left hand, and hold the hind leg steady by the hoof with your right hand (safety grip). Rest your right wrist on your knee. The knee is flexed 90°. You thus create a fixed point with your rightt hand, and your left hand pushes the hock away from you to create external rotation in the hip.

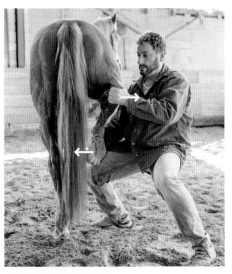

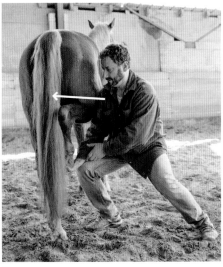

▼ INTERNAL ROTATION

Use the same grip as for external rotation, but this time your left hand pulls the hock toward you to obtain internal rotation.

▼ ADDUCTION + FLEXION

Starting in the neutral position, lift the flexed limb slightly, place your shoulder on the lateral aspect of the thigh, and gradually push with your shoulder, downward and toward the midline of the horse's body.

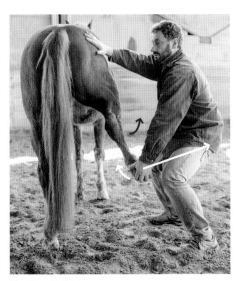

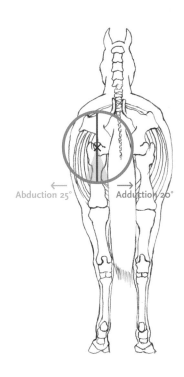

Abduction 25°   Adduction 20°

▼ ABDUCTION

Starting in the neutral position, bring the limb into flexion while very slowly rising to your feet. Place your right hand on the buttock at the level of the hip. Your left hand raises the hind leg laterally. The hip opens, and the spine adapts by rotating to the opposite side. Be careful not to force it; there is no point in taking this stretch especially far, and the horse may react defensively and push you back. The range of motion for abduction here is limited.

The spinal column

The spinal column stretches like a bridge between the support points of the shoulder girdle (anterior) and the pelvic girdle (posterior). For the cervical vertebrae, the biomechanics are different depending on whether you have a support in the mouth such as a bit, a halter on the head, or the head is free of all contact. Indeed, if the horse can lean on his jaw or head, this alters the fine postural organization of the cranio-cervical region. The jaw can then be viewed, mechanically speaking, as a third pair of supporting limbs. Its balance depends on the harmony of tension between the back muscles and the abdominals, and between the muscles of the girth and the jaw. There is no way to passively stretch the abdominal or paravertebral muscles. This would require lifting the stomach or pushing the back downward significantly, which would be quite difficult. You can engage in movements like these simply to stimulate the muscles, but it will not qualify as any kind of passive stretching test.

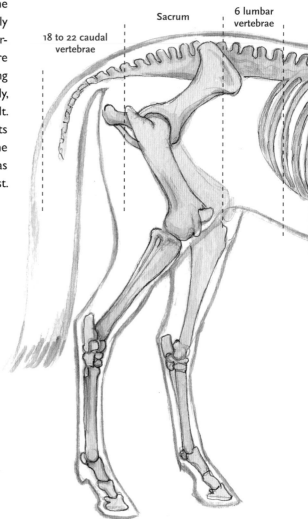

18 to 22 caudal vertebrae

Sacrum

6 lumbar vertebrae

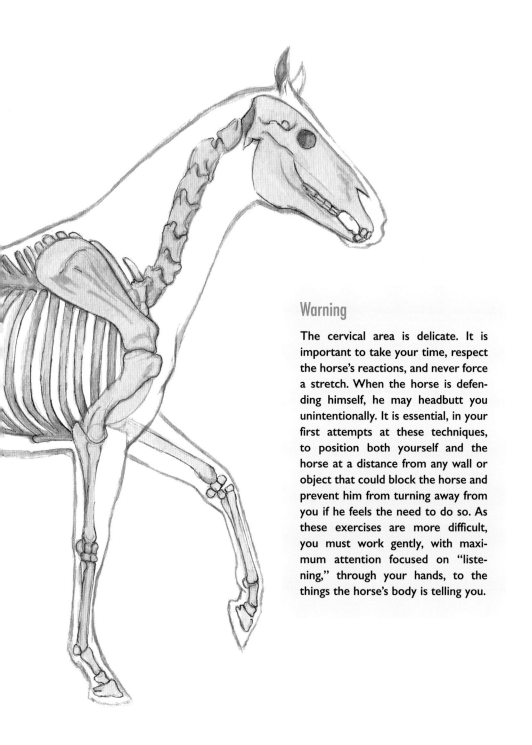

Warning

The cervical area is delicate. It is important to take your time, respect the horse's reactions, and never force a stretch. When the horse is defending himself, he may headbutt you unintentionally. It is essential, in your first attempts at these techniques, to position both yourself and the horse at a distance from any wall or object that could block the horse and prevent him from turning away from you if he feels the need to do so. As these exercises are more difficult, you must work gently, with maximum attention focused on "listening," through your hands, to the things the horse's body is telling you.

✦ Upper cervical mobilization

These tests are essential for any rider wishing to understand the behavior of her horse when he responds to rein aids. Above all, the issue here will be to try to determine whether any given problem needs to be solved through dentistry instead.

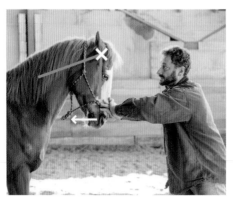

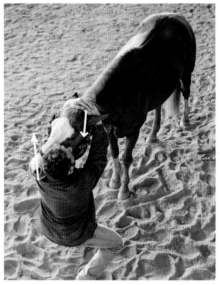

▼ **FLEXION**

Face the horse with your hands on the lower part of his nose. Push gently, focusing your movement to obtain mobilization between the head and the first cervical vertebra. You will feel all muscular resistance melt away, and perceive a flexion of the upper cervical vertebrae. Warning: some "locked" horses will turn their heads by compensating elsewhere instead of relaxing to the degree required for a release of tension here.

▼ **EXTENSION**

Place the horse's head on your shoulder and rest your head against his cheek. Your two hands come up and join behind his ears. Wait for the horse to relax, then accompany the descent of his neck with your hands, and adapt your position by shifting your weight to your back foot; the point of support for the horse on your shoulder should remain fixed.

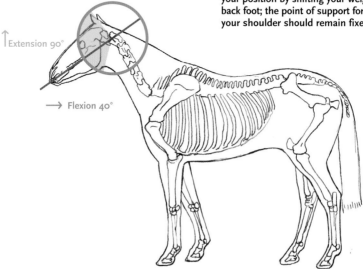

↑ Extension 90°

→ Flexion 40°

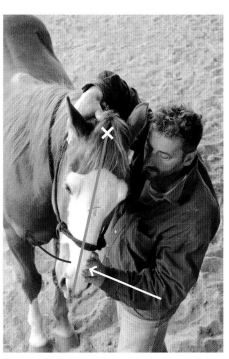

▼ ROTATION

Position yourself laterally on the side opposite the movement you will be looking for. One hand should grasp the nose, and the other, the first cervical vertebra. Push away from you with the hand on the nose, while the other hand supports and stabilizes the neck in a fixed position.

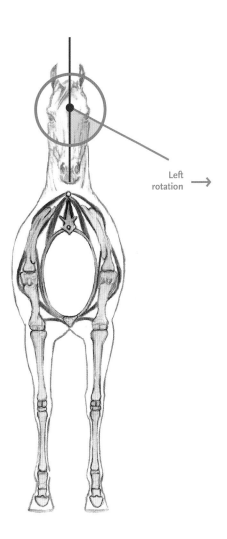

Left
rotation →

✦ Lower cervical mobilization

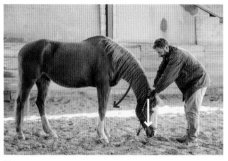

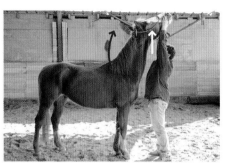

▼ FLEXION

Place both hands between the ears and accompany the descent of the horse's head.

▼ EXTENSION

Use the palms of your hands to laterally support the lower jaw, with the thumbs placed beneath it. Gently and gradually lift the horse's head and jaw (sometimes difficult to practice, depending on your height and the size of the horse) so that all the cervical vertebrae are extended vertically. At the limit of this stretch, you will notice a lowering of the withers.

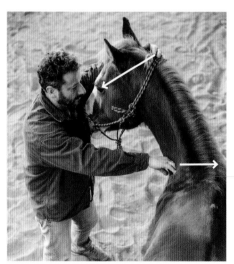

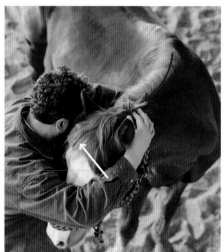

▼ TILT ANALOGOUS TO LATERAL ROTATION

Stand on the same side toward which you will be directing the horse's movement. Place one hand on the side of the horse's face further from you (do not grasp the halter, as your fingers might end up tangled there in the event of a defensive reaction), and calmly draw the horse's head towards you and around—toward the scapula to test the middle cervical vertebrae, or toward the flank to test the lower cervical vertebrae. Place your other hand on the middle or lower cervical vertebrae respectively.

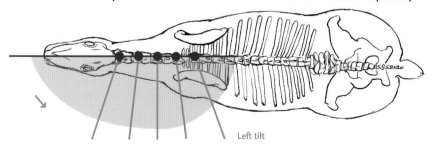

Left tilt

✦ Dorso-lumbar mobilization

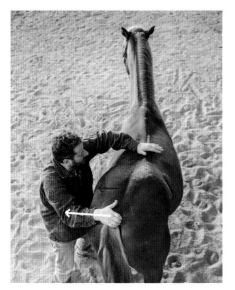

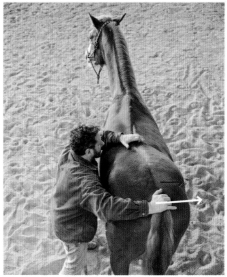

▼ LATERALITY

Stand against the horse's side. Place one hand flat on the root of the tail; this hand will be responsible for creating a lateral swaying motion. The other will move from vertebra to vertebra with each lateral motion, to assess the quality of the movement and to note any reactions. If you are positioned on the left side of the horse, this test will assess the limitations of mobility in left laterality. Switch sides to assess right laterality. With a little practice, you will be able to stay on the same side and test lateral capacity on both sides at once.

▼ LATERALITY

As shown above, your alternating movements should create a lateral ripple of the spine.

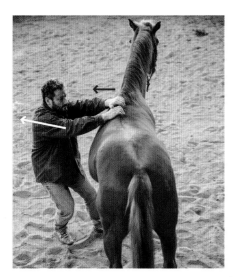

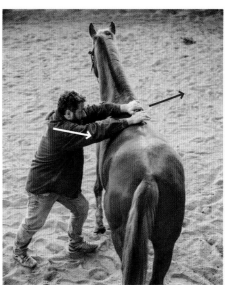

►▼ ROTATION OF THE WITHERS

Place your hands on the ridge of the withers and pull the horse toward you until you feel the horse's weight begin to lift off of the opposite foreleg. At this point, release the pull. Repeat, but this time by pushing until you feel the foreleg nearer to you lift, and then release the push.

✦ Tail mobilization

The coccygeal vertebrae extend from the sacrum and form the structure of the tail. The horse's tail is used for protection against insects, precise postural balance adjustments, and body language. Osteopathic lesions are frequent in this area, and often the cause of mechanical, visceral, and craniosacral "locking up" of the hindquarters. For all sports requiring a crupper, the ability of the horse to move the tail in a relaxed way is essential.

I offer you general movements here; you may have to adapt your approach in the event of a defensive reaction by the horse.

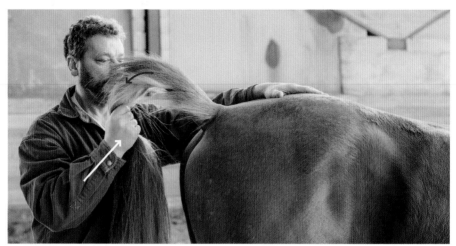

▼ FLEXION

Position yourself to one side of the horse. Gently lift the tail with one hand, and draw it up and over the horse's back, causing it to curve into a downward concave arc. This mobilization frequently generates a release of tension in the pelvis (triggers release of stool, urge to urinate, overall relaxation).

▲ EXTENSION

Position yourself to one side of the horse. Gently lift the tail with a slightly tugging hand, in such a way that it forms an upward concave arc. This mobilization frequently generates a release of tension in the pelvis (triggers release of stool, urge to urinate, overall relaxation).

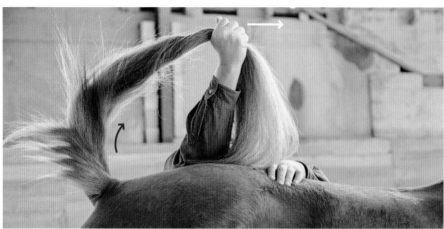

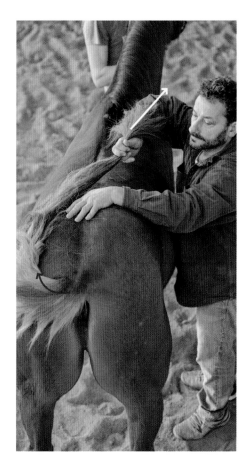

◄ LATERALITY

Start in the same position as for the previous test, with the tail extended. Then curve it to one side instead of upward, and lower it so that it rests along the buttock; repeat on the other side.

▼ TAIL TRACTION

To be practiced only with a relaxed horse whose behavior is trustworthy. Stand behind the horse, grasp the end of the tail with both hands with your arms outstretched, and lean back, using your body weight. The practitioner should look for the limit of the pulling movement of this stretch, and note the elasticity of the tissues involved. This stretch causes the horse's weight to settle more fully in his hindquarters. Then, the practitioner relaxes, and this should create a wave of mobility in the back. In a horse that is stuck in this area, the back will react as a single immobile unit, and the practitioner will not observe elasticity.

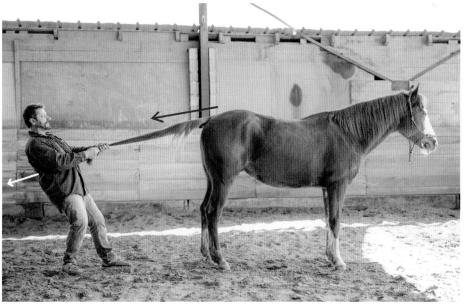

Test sequence for the forelegs

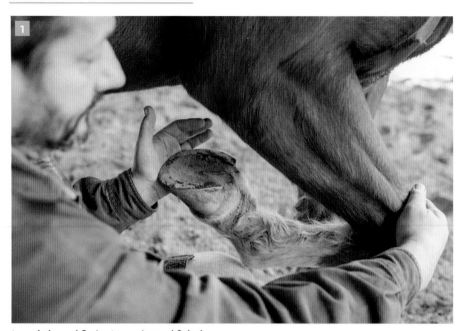

Interphalangeal flexion/extension and fetlock

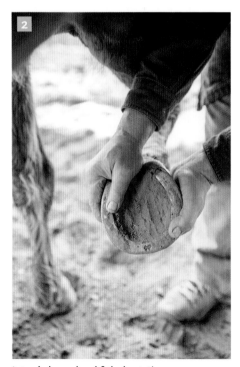

Interphalangeal and fetlock rotations

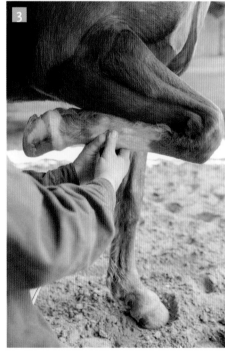

Knee flexion

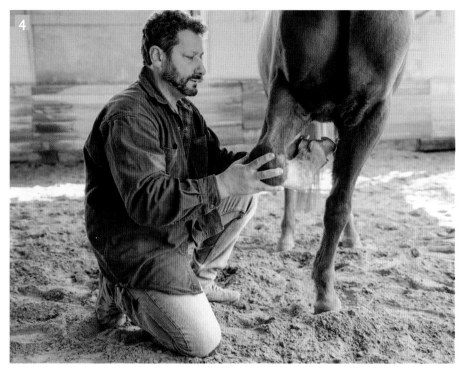

Knee rotation

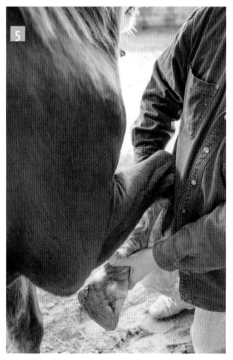

Elbow flexion

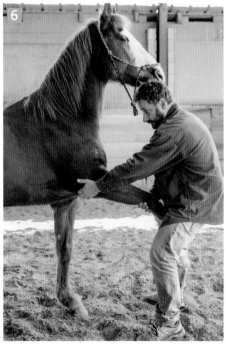

Shoulder extension

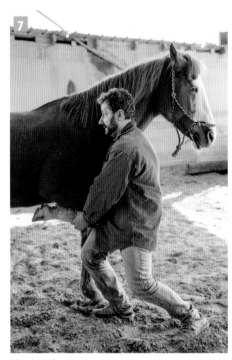

Shoulder flexion

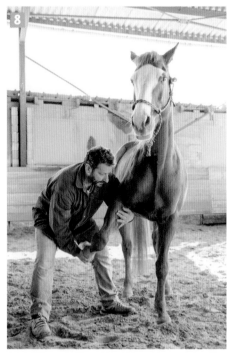

Shoulder abduction

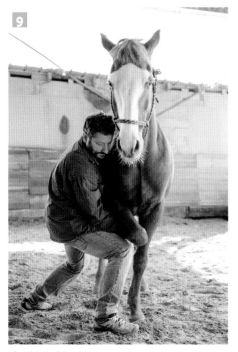

Shoulder adduction

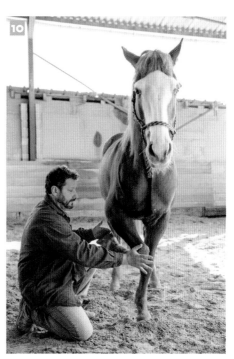

Internal rotation of the shoulder

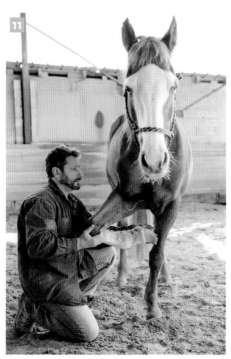

External rotation of the shoulder

Test sequence for the hind legs

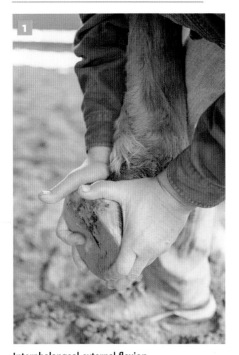

Interphalangeal external flexion

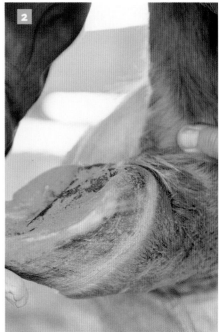

Flexion of the fetlock

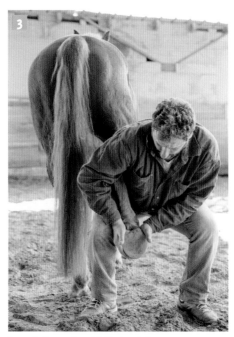

Interphalangeal and fetlock rotation

— STRETCH EXERCISES FOR HORSES

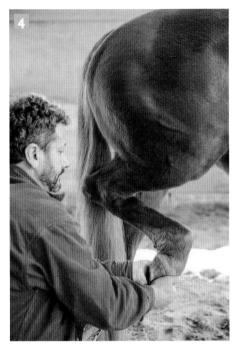

Hock flexion

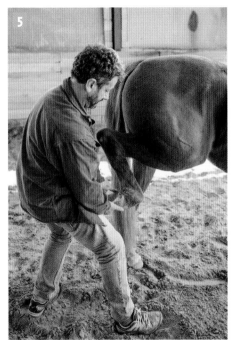

Stifle flexion

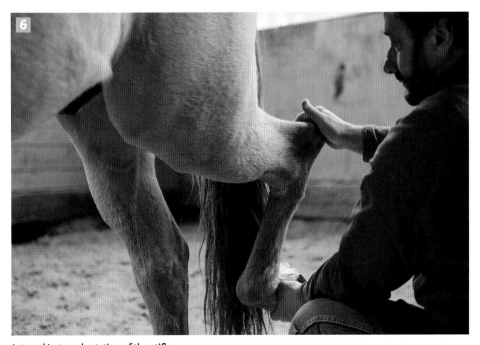

Internal/external rotation of the stifle

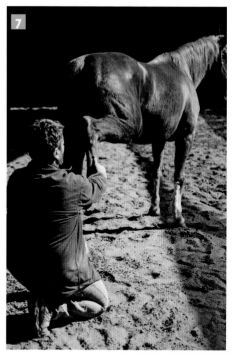

Extension of the hip

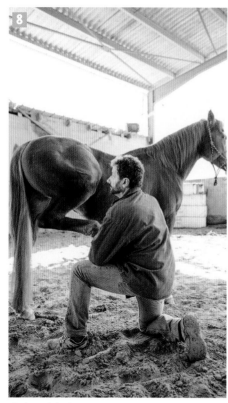

Flexion of the hip

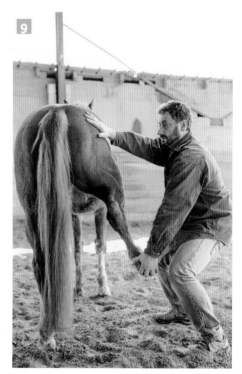

Hip abduction

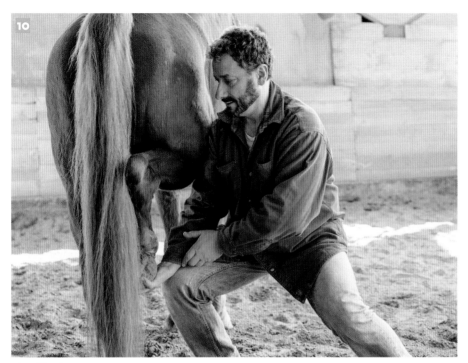

Hip adduction

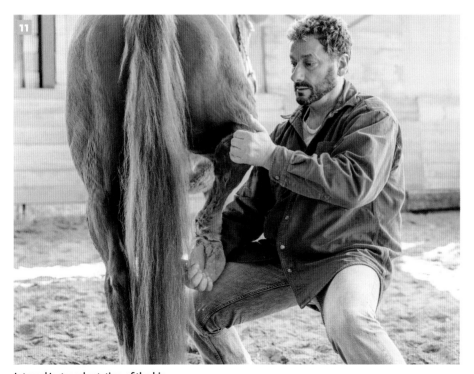

Internal/external rotation of the hip

Test sequence for the spinal column

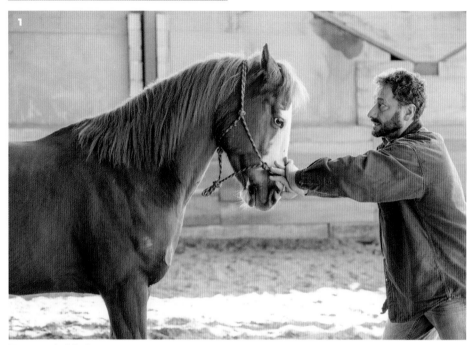

Upper cervical flexion

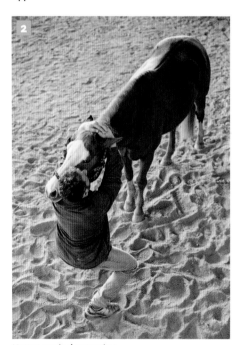

Upper cervical extension

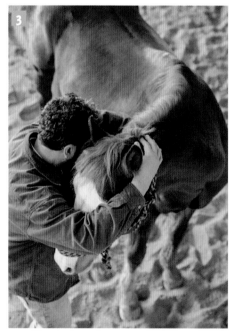

Stretching the lateroflexion muscles

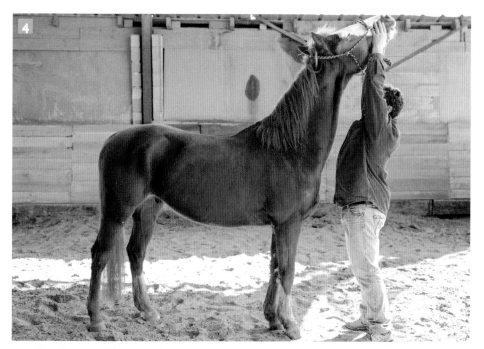

Stretching the cervical flexor muscles

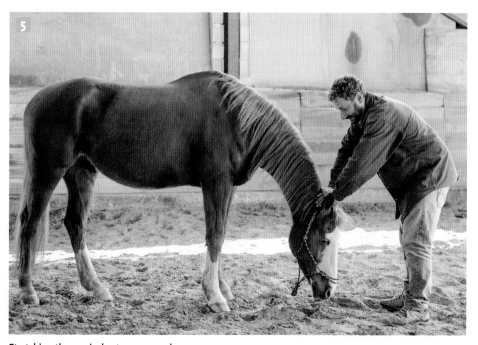

Stretching the cervical extensor muscles

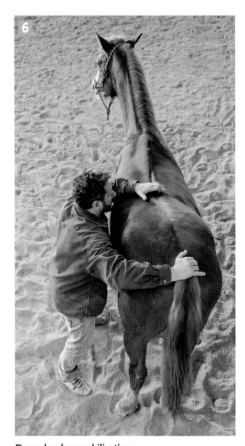

Dorso-lumbar mobilization

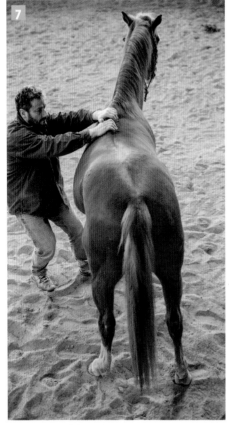

Mobilization of the withers

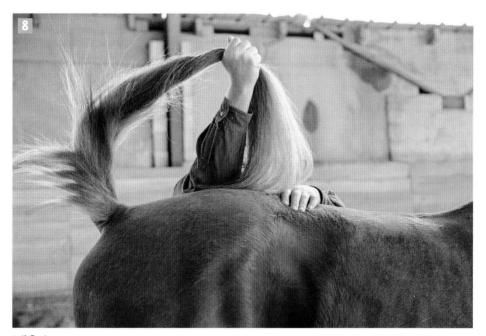

Tail flexion

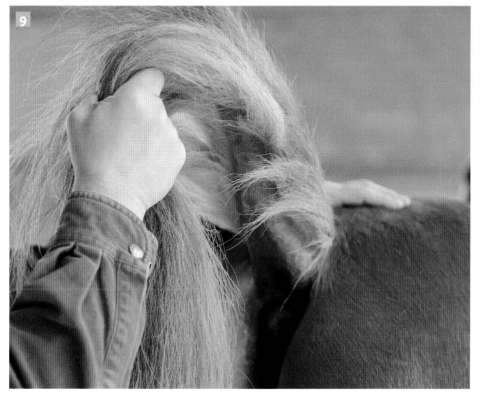

Tail extension

CHAPTER 6

MUSCLE CHAIN TESTS

These tests are always done from the neutral position, using the safety holds described in chapter 5. The practitioner allows the horse to explore, without force, his range of movement in one of four directions for each of the limbs. The foot should be kept as close to the ground as possible (an inch or two). At the slightest tension or defensive reaction, the practitioner must stop the test and remain within the comfort zone of the horse. It is always difficult to know whether a defensive reaction is due to a physical problem or a behavior problem. However, in general, a defensive reaction can probably be attributed to a physical issue if it is always triggered at the same place in the stretch and happens every time, as long as you have ruled out every possible issue with technique.

Tests for the anterior muscle chains

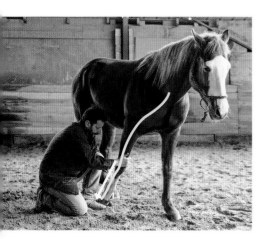

✦ Front and back muscle chains

Anterior muscle chain of the foreleg

Starting in the neutral position, with a safety grip on the hoof, offer a backward stretch, stopping at the slightest tension. The limb should be straight and the foot as close to the ground as possible. This stretch reaches up through the anterior muscles of the shoulder, all the way to certain lateral and flexor muscles of the neck. Pay close attention to the quality of the limit of this stretch, and any possible compensation.

Posterior muscle chain of the foreleg

Starting in the neutral position, with a safety grip on the hoof, offer a forward stretch, stopping at the slightest tension. The limb should be straight and the foot as close to the ground as possible. This stretch reaches up through the posterior muscles of the shoulder, all the way to certain lateral and extensor muscles of the withers. Pay close attention to the quality of the limit of this stretch, and any possible compensation.

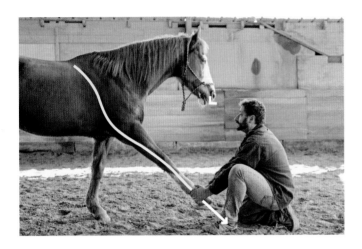

◆ Lateral chains
Internal chain of the foreleg

Starting in the neutral position, with a safety grip on the hoof, offer a stretch outward, away from the midline. This stretch is for the internal (pectoral) and fixator muscles of the scapula. Pay close attention to the quality of the limit of this stretch, and any compensation in the head or withers.

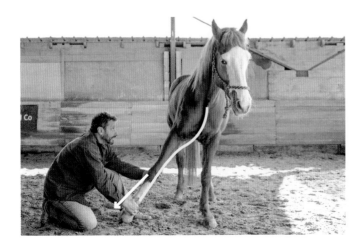

External chain of the foreleg

Starting in the neutral position, with a safety grip on the hoof, offer a stretch inward, toward the midline. The opposite limb, as the sole support for the forehand, cannot move out of the way, so it will be necessary to perform this stretch twice, exploring two ranges of motion: inward and forward, in front of the other foreleg; and inward and backward, behind the other foreleg. Most of the time, if you encounter difficulty in the forward/backward muscle chain tests, it will suffice to test the laterality with the easiest of the forward/backward chain movements. Position yourself opposite the limb you want to stretch. Grasp the back of the limb, and draw it forward, allowing the foot to skim the ground if it can (once for each of the two options, in front of the other foreleg [1] or in back [2]). Warning: be vigilant and gradual, because the shift in his weight here can throw the horse off balance toward you.

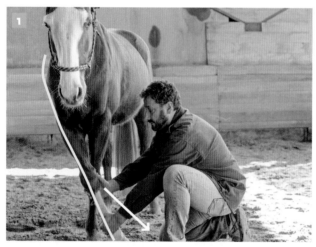

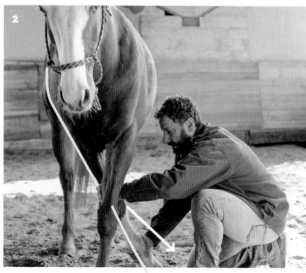

Tests for the posterior muscle chains

✦ Front and back muscle chains
Anterior muscle chain of the hind leg

Starting in the neutral position, with a safety grip on the hoof, offer a backward stretch. You will gradually feel any tension in the muscles in front of the hip and stifle release. At the limit of the elasticity of this stretch, there will be a mobilization of the iliac (tuber coxae) downwards, which tends to lead to an extension of the lumbar vertebrae, especially if the psoas muscle is contracted or retracted.

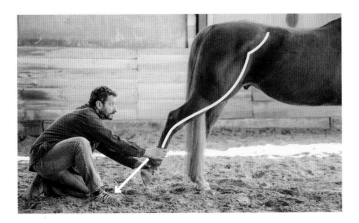

Posterior muscle chain of the hind leg

Starting in the neutral position, with a safety grip on the hoof, offer a forward stretch. You will gradually feel any tension in the muscles behind the hip and stifle release. At the limit of the elasticity of this stretch, there will be an upward mobilization of the iliac (tuber coxae), which tends to lead to flexion of the lumbar vertebrae.

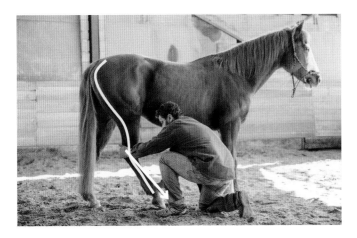

Tests for the muscle chains along the spine

✦ Inside chain

Starting in the neutral position, with a safety grip on the hind leg, offer a stretch outward, away from the midline. You will gradually feel any tension in the adductor muscles of the thigh release. Note any pelvic compensation. Sometimes the muscle lowers on the stretched side, and sometimes the horse shifts his weight to the other side, freeing musculoskeletal tension in the pelvis and lower back.

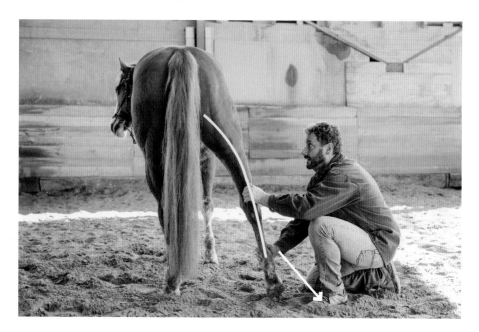

◆ Outside chain

The opposite limb, as the sole support for the hindquarters, cannot move out of the way, so it will be necessary to perform this stretch twice, exploring two ranges of motion: inward and forward, in front of the other hind leg; and inward and backward, behind the other hind leg. Most of the time, if you encounter difficulty in the forward/backward muscle chain tests, it will suffice to test the laterality with the easiest of the forward/backward chain movements.

Stand opposite the hind leg you want to stretch. Grasp the back of the limb, and draw it toward you, allowing the foot to skim the ground if it can (once for each of the two options, in front of the other hind leg [1] or in back [2]).

Warning: be vigilant and gradual, because the shift in his weight here can throw the horse off balance toward you.

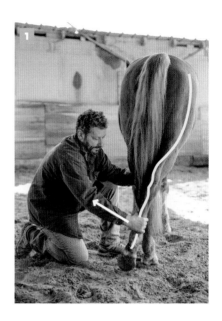

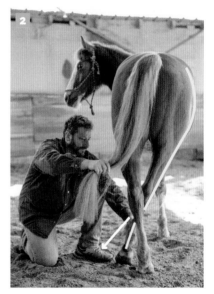

CHAPTER 7

EXAMPLES OF RELEASE THROUGH PASSIVE STRETCHING AND STIMULATION FOR ACTIVE STRETCHING

According to my method, after release by passive stretching, the horse must move: work in hand, at liberty, on the longe line, or under saddle. Active stimulation can be of great help to the rider. Once an area has been released by passive techniques, movement should be possible without reluctance or resistance. The use of a carrot (avoid the sugar lump) to achieve active neck stretches is well known and often used, and I recommend it. In this chapter, I offer you original and specific exercises to practice as well.

Stretching the postero-internal chain of the forelegs

This stretching is done when muscle chain tests show difficulty going backward and inward, and ease in going forward and outward. When you take hold of the foreleg, its neutral joint position is somewhat forward and outward. You're going to let the foreleg stretch out, and position yourself so that you feel balanced and comfortable. Your hands should grip the hoof by its tip; the foreleg will extend slightly in an outward direction. I continue this release until all tensions feel balanced. If the horse tries to draw his foreleg free of your grasp, slow his movement but do not prevent it, and then gently stretch again. If the foreleg is inclined inward, use the same strategy.

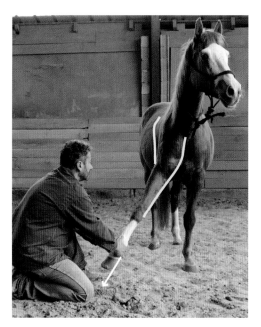

We see the release of the shoulder and scapula, and the pull on the withers, which sag. All the posterior shoulder muscles are stretched, with an elastic reaction at the limit of the stretch. These releases of the lateral muscle chains particularly help the horse during lateral movements, and also help unlock the withers.

> ### Tip
>
> Give a thirty-second massage to the muscles behind the shoulder blades on both sides before this stretch.

Stretching the antero-internal chain of the hind leg

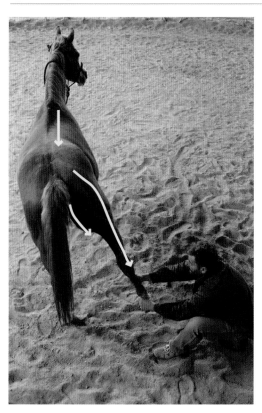

Take hold of the hind leg, and let it extend backward. Let the horse gradually surrender. When you feel that he is calm in this position, you can stand behind him. Always be alert and ready to move in the event of a strong reaction. You will gradually feel the tension in the muscles in front of the hip and stifle release. At the end of this release, there will be a mobilization of the iliac (tuber coxae) downwards, which tends to extend and open the lumbar vertebrae.

When the horse tries to draw his hind leg free of your grasp, slow down his movement, and assess what kind of reaction it is. It may be a slight contraction of the stretched muscles to test the sensation, or it may be that the horse has had enough and takes his leg back in a straightforward manner.

In either case, slow down his movement and then resume the test to determine where in the stretch that defensive reaction occurs. But this time, perhaps he'll let his leg go a little farther.... For safety, when the horse reacts this way, always move yourself to one side and keep your hand in contact with the hind leg.

> ## Tips
>
> - If you practice stretching as part of a warm-up before a work session (see chapters 3 to 5), a defensive contraction in reaction to this stretch will actually improve the relaxation of the muscles of the postero-external chain on the opposite side.
> - In order to relax a group of muscles, you have multiple options: you can stretch that group, contract the opposing muscles, or contract the same group of muscles on the opposite side.

Hula hoop

This exercise results in a general joint mobilization of either end of the horse's body. Areas of discomfort will be avoided so that the horse relaxes as he repeats this combination movement.

The hula-hoop is particularly recommended as:

- a general joint mobilization for daily maintenance for osteoarthritic horses;

- a pre-warm-up for very stiff horses;

- a desensitization routine to acclimatize young horses to complex movements on each limb;

- physical preparation for repetitive exertions planned for the same day (a jump-off, a trail ride, etc).

✦ Hula hoop for the hind legs

The hula hoop for the hind legs is broken down into three phases, illustrated by photographs 1, 2, and 3 (next page). Starting in the neutral position, using the left hand for a safety grip on the hoof, place your elbow on your left thigh to avoid supporting the weight of the horse with your back. Your right hand grasps the point of the hock. Positioning of the practitioner's feet is essential, and they should remain fixed in place during the exercise. The movement will be created by the practitioner drawing a horizontal circle with the pelvis—as if the practitioner were using an invisible hula hoop.

Thus, the joints of the horse's limb will move through all three spatial dimensions: forward/back, abduction/adduction, and internal rotation/external rotation.

✦ Hula hoop for the forelegs

As for the hind legs, the hula hoop for the forelegs breaks down into three stages (see next page for photos). Starting in the neutral position, grasp the horse's foreleg just above the knee with the right hand. Let the knee rest on the upper part of your thigh to avoid supporting the weight of the horse with your back.

The left hand grasps the internal bulb on the underside of the hoof to suspend the cannon bone horizontally without letting the hoof (or shoe) hit the elbow. Positioning of the practitioner's feet is essential, and they should remain fixed in place during the exercise. The practitioner's left foot should be positioned on a diagonal line with the left hind foot of the horse, and the right foot of the practitioner should be positioned just in front of the left front foot of the horse, in such a way that tracing from

Hula-hoop for the hind legs

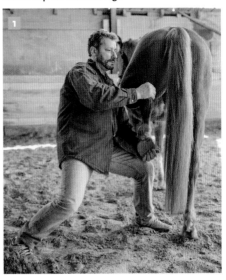

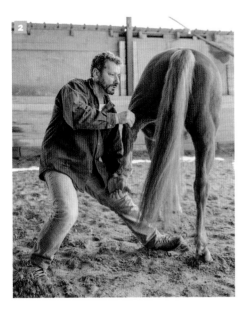

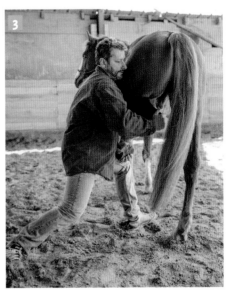

one of the practitioner's feet to the horse's left hind foot, and then to the practitioner's other foot, would yield an angle of approximately 90°. The movement will be created by the practitioner, drawing a horizontal circle with his own pelvis—as if using an invisible hula hoop. Thus, the joints of the horse's limb will move through all three spatial dimensions: forward/back, abduction/adduction, and internal rotation/external rotation.

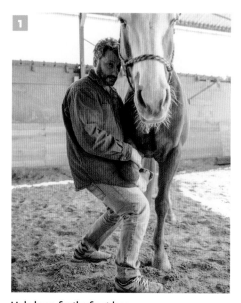 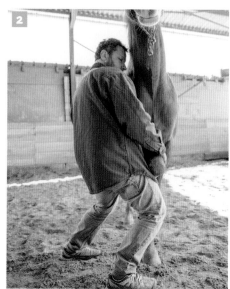

Hula-hoop for the front legs

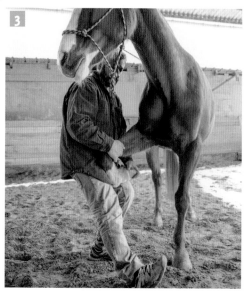

Stretching the cranio-cervical joint

Rest the horse's head on your shoulder and place both hands behind his ears. Wait without doing anything; the head is a difficult part of the body to release. Unless they suffer from severe upper neck tension problems, horses love this posture and often fall asleep.

This technique releases physical tension, but also emotional and mental tension in difficult horses. It frees the channel of the vagus nerve, eliminating many internal stresses.

The horse might neither react defensively nor give in fully to this stretch. However, it's important to realize that by letting his head be guided down or taking away any of the weight of his head, he is beginning to let go.

Next, feel him release in extension. Begin to accompany him in lengthening into the stretch. After 5 minutes, he relaxes entirely and falls asleep.

Sometimes, when significant tension is released, the horse's cervical vertebrae release both laterally and up/down. The technique of listening through feel remains the same: stay with the horse until his reactions stop. This is the only technique that allows a deep relaxation of the horse that can free him from old traumatic memories, embedded in his tissues and his behavior.

Above and beyond an exceptional shared experience of the horse finally letting go fully, this test also provides information on the animal's most deeply rooted behavior.

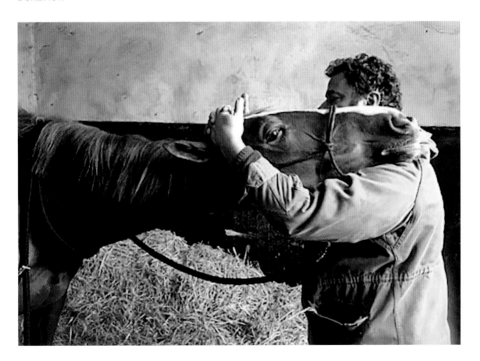

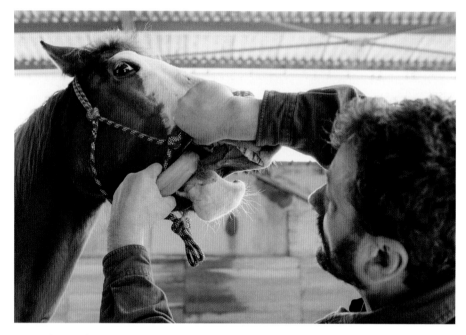

Stretching the tongue

Position yourself to one side of the horse, and place the back of one hand at mouth level under the halter; the other hand will gently grasp the tongue. Wait for the horse to relax, and then slowly, gently draw his tongue out of his mouth and place it in the hand holding the halter. The horse will relax. Hold the tongue stretch for about 30 seconds on each side, and assess whether one side feels stretchier than the other. Once you know which side is which, always start the stretch on the easier side. The horse should respond to the stretch sooner or later by swallowing, which works the stretch up to the larynx. Take advantage of this test to observe the color of the mucus membranes in the mouth, the color of the blood in the veins located under the tongue, any scars on the jaw and tongue, and the behavior displayed by the horse in this context. Having the tongue grasped is unusual, and can be stressful for horses that have had mouth problems. This is why you should be very gradual and gentle with this stretch; don't turn to force if the horse expresses reluctance. Desensitization is essential, and can be a solution to many mechanical and behavioral problems in the horse under saddle. Stretching the tongue sometimes causes a cough, which should be noted on your observation sheet. Warning: never use force to counter a defensive reaction from the horse, and always hold the tongue with the hand holding the halter.

This exercise is very informative for the rider in terms of both the mechanical action and the behavior of the horse when his mouth is touched or manipulated. Sometimes desensitization of the tongue is necessary, as this area is rarely explored in this way. One potential defensive reaction is bringing the tongue to the side, common in cases of "step mouth."

Active stretching using the "Masticator" activator

This activator stimulates chewing, salivation, and active mobilization of the jaw and upper cervical vertebrae. It is a valuable tool for horses with delicate mouths. Its use serves as a pre-warm-up to encourage connection with the mouth. The rider then works her horse as usual with the bit of her choice.

I also make use of this tool after treatment, when dental leveling is necessary. It will maintain osteopathic regulation before the dentist arrives. By encouraging a fairly broad dynamic movement, the muscles are actively stretched, and relaxation takes place after a few days. In horses with severe occlusion problems or temporomandibular joint mobility dysfunction, this activator can help improve the function of the horse's mouth.

Protocol: Put in the mouth 10 to 15 minutes before work, and 5 minutes after. Sometimes the horse stops chewing; if this happens, put a little honey (or other favored flavoring) on the activator. This exercise is complementary to the tongue stretch.

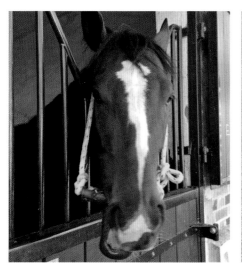 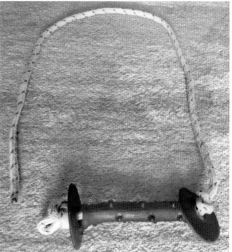

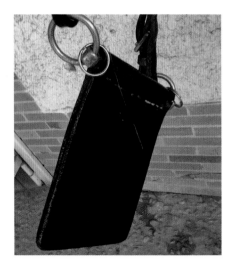 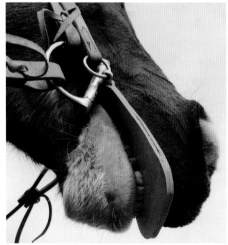

"Equilibrator" dental occlusion orthosis

The principle of this orthosis is to improve the quality of interdental contact (occlusion). The plastic or leather flap improves the mobility of each tooth, which, when the bite is poor, tends to be blocked or changed. Wearing this orthosis, postural regulation takes place very quickly, because the support of the Equilibrator elevates the incisors, and consequently relieves the pressure on the molars and changes the mechanical stresses on the joints of the jaw. This device can also be used as a differential test to find out whether jaw dysfunction is due to a tooth imbalance problem or temporomandibular joint imbalance syndrome.

When the horse always leans on the same side of the mouth, this orthosis can be a good solution while waiting for tissues to release after manipulation, or after leveling of the teeth by the dentist.

For your purposes, it is best to have one hard plastic flap and another made of leather or rubber. Horses' reactions to hardness can be very different. For more than twenty years, I have recommended wearing it while waiting for a dentist's treatment, as well as to provide diagnostic evidence distinguishing between behavioral and mechanical problems in connection with the head. This device is very useful for horses with osteoarthritis of the jaw also. To be worn by the horse from time to time during the week, adapting as needed to develop the most suitable protocol.

Protocol: Put in the mouth by attaching the flap without tension, so it will not pull at the corners of the mouth.

Active stretching and stimulation

Active stretching consists of stimulating the horse so he moves in a given direction on request, from either touch, or a carrot or apple (avoid more refined sugars, which are not good for his health), in such a way as to elicit the desired movement.

The touch generates a reflex reaction, and requires the practitioner's know-how to guide the direction and orientation of the stretch. The reaction is brief (about one second long).

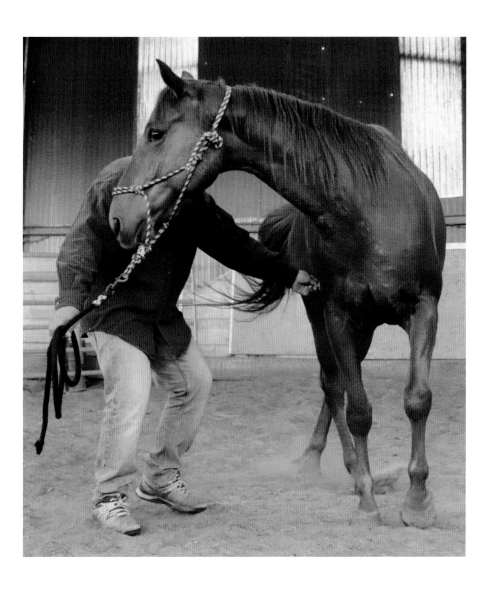

The carrot enables a voluntary, non-reflex reaction from the horse. By positioning him correctly, and provided your horse wants to bite the carrot badly enough, you will obtain a stretch of 10 seconds or more in the direction most useful for the rehabilitation, toning, or post-traumatic desensitization of the horse.

This kind of dynamic stretching is wonderfully complementary to the passive stretching described previously. It is a needed intermediary stage between the very specific rehabilitation of passive care, and the rehabilitation and readaptation facilitated by physiotherapeutic treatment before a horse who has suffered injury can resume work under saddle. Once all three of these stages of rehabilitation have been completed, a horse can be ridden, resume normal work, and continue his development as an athlete or his daily life.

Here are three examples of very useful active stretches that can be achieved with carrots:

- cervico-dorsal flexion;

- lateral cervico-dorsal flexion;

- cervical laterality.

✦ Cervico-dorsal flexion

The practitioner takes a carrot in each hand and stands to one side of the horse. The hand closer to the head will begin the movement.

The practitioner squats down, passes the other hand between the forelegs, and draws the horse's attention with the second carrot, so that he stretches his head down and back between his forelegs until he reaches the limit of elasticity that will tend to raise the withers. Try to hold this stretch for at least ten seconds, and repeat the exercise four times. Note any compensations he might show at the end of the stretch. This gives us very useful information for mounted work to come, and allows us to avoid reinforcing these compensations. A full stretch of the entire dorsal chain of the back takes place at the limit of this stretch.

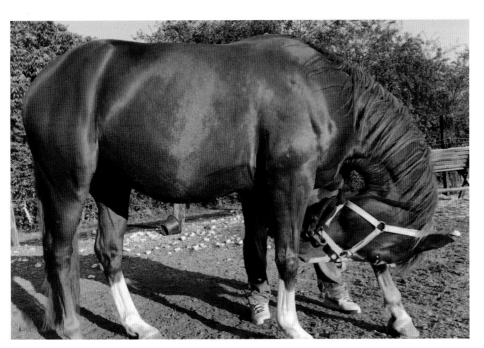

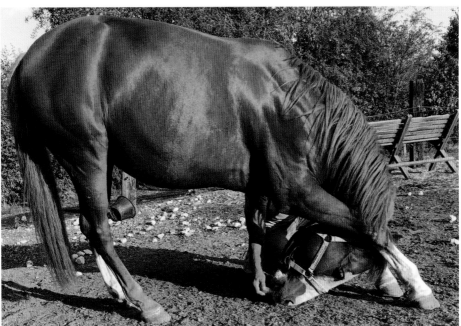

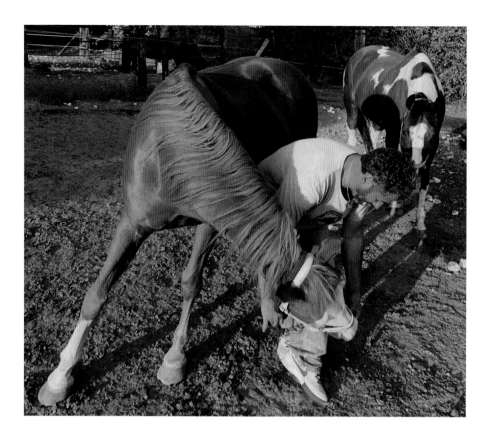

✦ Lateral cervico-dorsal flexion

To obtain laterality and flexion of the cervical and upper vertebrae, the practitioner should be positioned with the back at the level of the left scapula of the horse, and, with a carrot held in the left hand, attracts the attention of the horse. The practitioner then gradually bends to lower the carrot as close to the ground as possible. The horse will wrap himself around the practitioner to follow. Thus, the upper cervical vertebrae remain in extension or neutral position; the middle and lower cervicals and the first dorsals will reverse their natural curvature towards flexion, stretching all muscle chains of extension and opposite laterality. The positioning of the practitioner between the left side and the head of the horse as the horse tries to catch the carrot is very important. It allows the practitioner to keep the horse from moving his feet, and thus forces the horse to use largely laterality and flexion, by transferring weight from the forelegs.

This stretch mobilizes the shoulder blades and improves laterality in both directions at the withers.

✦ Cervical laterality

The goal of this active stretch is to obtain laterality from a neutral so-called "anatomical" position of the horse. The practitioner takes a carrot in each hand. With the left hand, the horse is invited to come and get the carrot, and then both hands are brought together when the horse's head is at the level of the thorax, to keep the movement oriented for neutral laterality that constitutes neither extension nor flexion. The practitioner will then note any compensations the horse may have during this movement, when he is at the limit of active elasticity.

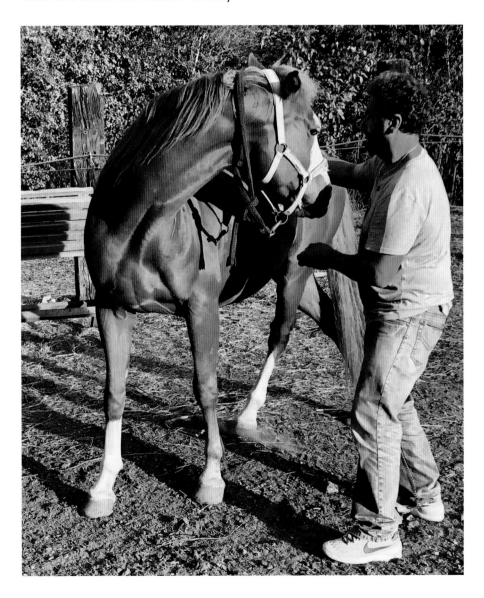

Depending on the scenario, the movement may be finished by raising the hands to guide the horse into an extension, or lowering the hands to create laterality with flexion close to the flank.

If the horse is really flexible, his body will form a nice even curve. If the horse is stiff, he will tend to move his buttocks and turn in a single inflexible unit to get the carrot. In this latter case, we should always start the next iteration of the stretch on the easier side—that is to say, the more flexible side, where the horse can bend instead of turning with the buttocks. Afterwards, return to the stiffer side. With very flexible horses, it is not uncommon for the horse to be able to reach his own croup, or even further, and collect the carrot.

Stimulation of active flexion mobilization of the thoraco-lumbar spine

Stand behind the horse, after making sure he is willing to accept you touching him on the buttocks. With a plastic needle cap in each hand (or with your fingernails), you will stimulate the horse's glutes and induce a general flexion reaction in the thoracolumbar spine. This is both a test to assess the sensitivity level of the horse's back, and a way to release minor tension in the horse's back. If the horse's back collapses as a result of this stimulation, on one or both sides, this indicates likely sciatica-type pain. You will often hear crackles of joint decompression. Do this stimulation three to four times, gently, without force, taking note of the horse's reactions. The movement obtained will give you information about the rebound potential of your horse.

Stimulation of left lateral mobilization and active flexion of the thoraco-lumbar spine

In the stall, I advise you to position yourself on the side of the horse with the easiest lateral movement. Walk the horse forward with one hand on the halter, and the other offering stimulation with a plastic needle cap (or other object) under the horse's stomach to achieve flexion and laterality of the spine. Make a dozen circles on each side. This exercise is an excellent opportunity to obtain flexion and laterality of the spine behind the often hypersensitive or immobile withers, which are commonly "locked up" due to a poorly fitted or poorly positioned saddle.

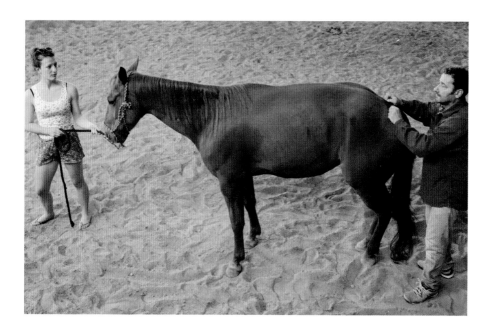

In an anatomical configuration with spinal processes that are too close together, this stimulation helps the horse re-engage, without weight, tension, or strain, in a movement that has been impossible for him for some time, and it can serve as mechanical and mental rehabilitation after osteopathic manipulation or other medical care. This stimulation should be done before and after a work session.

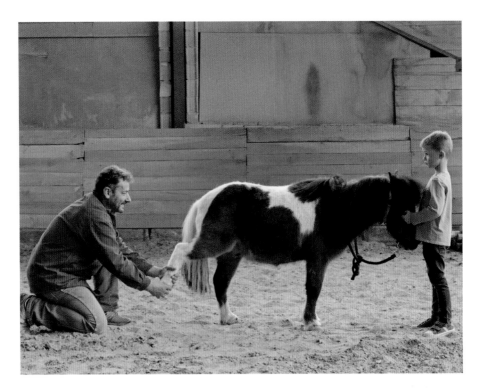

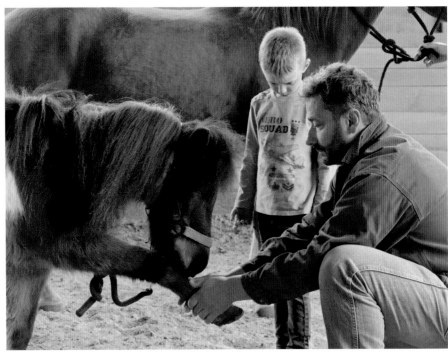

— STRETCH EXERCISES FOR HORSES

CONCLUSION

Whatever the size of the horse, the stretching technique remains the same; it is only your ability to adapt that will truly come into play to determine the outcome of a stretching session.

The practice of stretching is part of a mindful approach to preventative healthcare. It allows you to listen attentively to the messages of your horse's tissues, and thus to better understand his qualities and his faults, giving you the opportunity to plan his progress and yours appropriately. This unique method, allowing an effective analysis of the physical, energetic, emotional, and mental capacities of the horse, will make the management and progression of training more precise. It is a process that involves commitment of time, energy, and mental investment, and leads to exceptional partnership between you and your horse.

The same sequences and movements will be repeated at each session, and yet no two sessions will ever be the same. The resistances discovered will be those of the moment, so it is a matter of capturing them, listening to them, and releasing them. Remember that your hands must be relaxed, reassuring, and at one with the horse, in order for you to fully explore until you feel your horse's tensions loosen deep within his body. The more experience you have, the more refined your sense of feel will be, and the more confidence you will have in your assessments. All riders who have come to learn about neuro-muscular stretching report to me that they ride their horses differently, using the principles described in this method.

The various case studies published on the benefits of my neuro-muscular stretching method demonstrate its effectiveness in improving recovery after exertion, flexibility, muscle relaxation, and mental balance, improving performance over the season and lowering veterinary costs.

Remember to provide horses with a living environment that allows them sufficient space in which to move and gives them the opportunity to connect to nature.

And take heart! Have courage; dare to use your own two hands, to discover the subtleties of touch, to activate your horse's cellular release without any risk. Trust yourself and give your horse the gift of true freedom to use his body fully: he will love it.

Remember that *fair riding* results from balance in the horse-and-rider partnership, physically, energetically, emotionally, and mentally. The horse plays the role of emotional regulator. If you manage your stress, so will he, and magic will happen. This profound awareness will allow you both to perform better.

Working with horses is a genuinely personal job; it means taking the risk of questioning yourself in order to move forward on your life's path.

Thank you to the horses for what they bring us.

ACKNOWLEDGMENTS

I express my gratitude to all the people who have taught me what they know about listening and the art of touch—the riders, coaches, and all my students who trust me and thanks to whom my techniques evolve. I would particularly like to thank in various ways:

- Dominique Giniaux, Marvin Cain, Stuart McGregor, Bernard Achou, Julien Carayon, Stéphanie Penot, and Carl Nafzger;

- Adamo Walti and his horse Diamond, and Tracy and his pony, who posed for the photographs;

- Morgane Vallé and Maurine and Constance Boudard for taking the photographs.

Your thoughts interest me! Please write to me at this address:

Jean-Michel BOUDARD
Offices of Jean-Michel Boudard
27, Avenue Mac MAHON
75017 Paris

boudard-osteo-paris.com

You can find instructional videos on my YouTube channel.

INDEX

Page numbers in *italics* indicate illustrations.